THE
ARTHRITIS
CURE

P9-DDB-329

THE
ARTHRITIS
CURE

THE MEDICAL MIRACLE
THAT CAN HALT, REVERSE,
AND MAY EVEN <u>CURE</u> OSTEOARTHRITIS

REVISED EDITION

Revised Edition by
Jason Theodosakis, M.D., M.S., M.P.H., F.A.C.P.M.,
and **Sheila Buff**

Original Edition by Jason Theodosakis, M.D., M.S., M.P.H.,
Brenda Adderly, M.H.A., and Barry Fox, PH.D.

ST. MARTIN'S GRIFFIN ☙ **NEW YORK**

To those who can turn a challenge
into a worthy mission.
—Jason Theodosakis, M.D.

THE ARTHRITIS CURE, REVISED EDITION. Copyright © 2004 by Jason Theodosakis, M.D. All rights reserved. Printed in the United States of America. No part of this book may be used or reproduced in any manner whatsoever without written permission except in the case of brief quotations embodied in critical articles or reviews. For information, address St. Martin's Press, 175 Fifth Avenue, New York, N.Y. 10010.

Illustrations copyright © 1997 by Jackie Aher

www.stmartins.com

ISBN 0-312-32789-7

First Revised Edition: January 2004

10 9 8 7 6 5 4 3 2 1

Acknowledgments

To my family for their patience and understanding, Jessica Galow for her support and motivation, Dr. Lisa Sumner for her editorial comments in the chapter on rheumatic diseases, Sheila Buff for being such a joy to work with, and Heather Jackson for constantly moving this project forward.

Important Note to Readers

The material in this book is for informational purposes only. It is not intended to serve as a prescription for you, or to replace the advice of your medical doctor. Please discuss all aspects of the Arthritis Cure with your physician *before* beginning the program. If you have any medical conditions, or are taking any prescription or nonprescription medications, see your physician before beginning the program or altering or discontinuing your use of medications.

The fact that a Web site or another source is listed in this book as a potential source of information does not mean that my coauthor, publisher, or I endorse any of the information it may provide or recommendations it may make. Likewise, the fact that my own Web site is listed does not mean that my coauthor or publisher endorse any of the information it may provide or recommendations it may make.

Nothing in the title or content of this book is intended to suggest that the use of the recommended supplements will fully eradicate osteoarthritis. The evidence, carefully presented in this book, substantiates that the nutritional supplements recommended are frequently effective, even for long periods. Even so, I offer no guarantee that *every* individual will benefit from this program.

To protect their privacy, pseudonyms have been used for the individual patients mentioned in this book, and in some instances minor biographical details about them have been altered.

Contents

A Word from Dr. Theodosakis

Why do I even mention the word *cure* in the same sentence with "a chronic condition"?

I use the word *cure* to mean the partial or complete relief of symptoms of osteoarthritis. I have developed and used the program described in this book with my patients and have seen impressive results. Some of these patients had been unable to get relief from, or could not tolerate, traditional therapies. Some remain symptom-free—even those who are no longer taking the supplements. The safety and effectiveness of the supplements discussed in this book have now been verified in long-term, human clinical trials. As you read this book and decide with your doctor whether to use the supplements, you should keep in mind the following:

- Osteoarthritis is truly a variable condition—that is, two people with the same stage of cartilage damage may have different symptoms and respond differently to treatment.
- If your cartilage is worn down completely to the bone, your chances of cure are surely remote. However, the program described in this book may still offer you dramatic relief, help you postpone surgery (sometimes for years), and help you to avoid the dangers of traditional pain relievers and traditional treatment. The program is a safer and perhaps more effective treatment alternative than most standard therapies.
- The previous edition of *The Arthritis Cure* introduced the public to the benefits of glucosamine and chondroitin. This edition expands on these supplements, introduces a new disease-modifying agent, and discusses issues of potency and purity.
- Sadly, about 80 percent of the glucosamine and chondroitin products on the market have fallen short on ingredients or have significant quality concerns. Therefore, if you have not experi-

enced success, it is possible that you used the wrong product. My aim is to correct this so you're given the best chance possible to improve your health.

- Some cases of secondary osteoarthritis are reversible, and there are other medical conditions that mimic the symptoms of osteoarthritis. By treating the underlying medical condition, the arthritic symptoms may disappear forever. Therefore, a thorough diagnosis is critical to determine the best treatment. Don't just treat your symptoms, get an accurate diagnosis first.

Foreword

The field of medicine is a fascinating mixture of science, art, and philosophy. Since time and resources are limited, often business and political issues determine medical policies, practices, and beliefs. I knew these issues, not the science, would be the limiting factors to the acknowledgement and later acceptance of what was considered to be a radical idea—the first treatment that could alter the course of the common and painful disease osteoarthritis (OA).

Performing and publishing clinical studies is key to the advancement of medicine. Relaying this information to the public and to the medical profession in an understandable manner is equally important, however. Over 2,200 biomedical journals are available, and more studies are published every few months than the average physician could possibly read in an entire career. Too much sound research and good information simply never make it to the people who need it most.

As a professor and lecturer, my talent is my ability to relay information. My strategy to accelerate the acceptance of this superior treatment approach for OA was to educate the public first, then focus on the medical and scientific communities, and finally reach the old guard—the medical policymakers.

In medicine, old, long-used treatments are sometimes slow to change, especially if those involved in fostering this change are politically or financially motivated to maintain the status quo. In the end, however, science wins out, and the new replaces the old.

This has been the case for almost all major advances in medicine, a trend that will continue far into the future. My motivation to accelerate this change in the case of osteoarthritis was not simply out of the great public need. I hoped to change arthritis treatment because the traditional treatments are, in my opinion, a violation of the physician's Hippocratic oath to "Do no harm."

The traditional approach to treating people with OA not only just covers up the symptoms without addressing the root causes, but leads to significant suffering of its own. Over 16,000 patients are dying each year just trying to find relief from the unrelenting pain of arthritis.

We know that the use of just one of the nine steps outlined in this book—the supplements glucosamine, chondroitin and ASU—can dramatically reduce or eliminate the need for most people to rely on prescription and over-the-counter drugs for pain relief. The treatment program as a whole is likely to save several thousand lives each year in the United States alone. This has far exceeded my career hope to make a difference as one member of the millions involved in health care.

Although this is a popular health book, I don't like to be called an "alternative" physician. My rigorous medical training gives me a solid grounding in conventional medicine and a great respect for the miracles it can perform. However, all medical practices and principles are alternative at some point, until accepted into the norm. With millions using part or all of the treatment program to find relief from arthritis pain, the Arthritis Cure is well on the path to becoming the standard first-line treatment. This updated and revised edition includes all the wonderful new information and supporting studies that have become available since the first edition of the book appeared in 1997.

Jason Theodosakis,
M.D., M.S., M.P.H., F.A.C.P.M

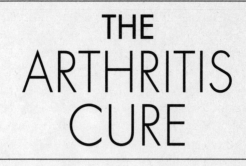

THE
ARTHRITIS
CURE

—1—
CAN OSTEOARTHRITIS BE CURED?

What is osteoarthritis?

Why is cartilage the focal point of the disease?

What are the symptoms of osteoarthritis and which joints are affected?

What causes osteoarthritis?

Who is affected by osteoarthritis?

What is the difference between osteoarthritis and rheumatoid arthritis?

How is osteoarthritis diagnosed?

What substances are being used to cure osteoarthritis?

It starts with a little stiffness in your right knee. Nothing to worry about. Then you notice that the pain is getting worse, that you sometimes have trouble walking and jogging really hurts. Or perhaps there's a bit of "morning stiffness" in your hip, and it's a chore to go up and down the stairs. Something has to be done about this—you've got a life to live! You visit your doctor.

The examination is routine, hardly more than a bit of probing. As you lie on the examination table in a paper dressing gown, the doctor moves your leg up and down and from side to side. "Does it hurt when I move your leg this way?" she asks. When you nod, she says, "Hmm. I'd like to order an X ray."

The X ray shows an uneven narrowing of the joint space between the bones of your right knee. Frowning as she studies the X ray, the doctor pronounces the diagnosis: "You have osteoarthritis. You know, 'wear and tear' arthritis. Osteoarthritis really starts ten to twenty years before you notice the first symptoms."

"Why didn't you tell me twenty years ago about this so I could have stopped playing tennis on those hard courts and weekend football with my friends? What should I do now?" you ask anxiously.

"Take aspirin or ibuprofen for the pain," she answers reassuringly. "And don't overexercise the knee."

"But how did I get it?"

"Osteoarthritis is practically inevitable," your doctor replies. "Almost everyone your age has it. The problem is the cartilage, which protects the ends of the bones. It's wearing away, and without that cartilage to keep your bones apart, they're grinding together, causing the pain and stiffness. That's essentially all there is to osteoarthritis. We can take care of the pain, up to a point, but unfortunately, there's nothing else we can do about it."

The Number-One Cause of Disability and Chronic Pain

Arthritis causes symptoms and problems in nearly 70 million Americans, or about one in every three adults.[1] As the population ages and develops more obesity, diabetes, and joint injuries, this number will only increase. Right now, about 60 percent of Americans over age 65, or some 21 million people, have arthritis. That number is expected to double over the next few decades—by 2030, the number of older adults in the U.S. with arthritis or chronic joint pain will top 41 million.

Arthritis doesn't just cause minor discomfort—it's the leading cause of disability among U.S. adults. In fact, arthritis accounts for some 17 percent of all disability nationwide. That's well ahead of heart disease, which is about 11 percent of all disability.[2] Arthritis now limits everyday activities for more than 7 million Americans; by 2020, this number will increase to perhaps 12 million as the population ages.

Disability from arthritis creates huge costs for those affected, their families, and the nation's economy. Each year, arthritis results in about

$15 billion of direct medical costs for 44 million outpatient visits and 750,000 hospitalizations. The estimated total cost to society, including lost work productivity, is about $83 billion every year.[3]

Arthritis is not one disease, but a group of diseases whose common threads are that they cause pain, inflammation, limited movement, and destruction of the joints. Three out of five arthritis sufferers are under age 65—arthritis is not a disease just of the elderly.

Though there are more than a hundred diseases that affect the musculoskeletal system, the most common form by far is osteoarthritis. In fact, osteoarthritis is more common than all other forms of arthritis combined. Because osteoarthritis is one of the forms of arthritis that becomes more common as we age, many people just assume it's a normal part of aging, that pain in the joints is like gray hair or wrinkles, something we should expect. But in fact, osteoarthritis usually starts in middle age or even earlier, often many years before a person first notices symptoms.

In a joint afflicted with osteoarthritis, the cartilage that covers and cushions the ends of the bones degenerates, allowing bones to rub together. In addition, bone spurs and cysts may develop and the structures around the joint, such as tendons, ligaments, and muscles, may become strained, inflamed, and painful. The major symptom of osteoarthritis is pain; inflammation (swelling, redness, and warmth in the area) is usually a problem only later in the course of the disease. Often, however, osteoarthritis can occur without pain—the main symptom is that the affected joints become stiff and less flexible. Some people don't notice this loss of range of motion, because it tends to occur very gradually. For instance, you may not be able to turn your head to the side as easily as you could in the past while trying to back up your car. Even if you don't have any neck pain, this could be a sign of osteoarthritis in the upper spine.

Up until recently, doctors in the United States thought that osteoarthritis was incurable. That's why the commonly prescribed treatment is strictly palliative, designed only to relieve the pain without addressing the true causes of the disease or the condition of the joints. For mild cases, doctors prescribe painkillers such as acetaminophen (Tylenol®) or nonsteroidal anti-inflammatory drugs (NSAIDs) such as aspirin or ibuprofen (Motrin®, Advil®). Steroid injections such as corti-sone and opiates (narcotics) are reserved for the more resistant cases. Unfortunately, the painkillers and anti-inflammatories have problems. They temporarily relieve pain, but in the long run they simply cover up the symptoms while the disease progresses further. These drugs have side effects that range from the annoying to the downright danger-ous—each year, thousands of people die from the adverse effects of anti-inflammatories, acetaminophen, and steroids. To add insult to injury, recent research suggests that nonsteroidal anti-inflammatories, including the new COX-2 inhibitors (such as Vioxx®, Celebrex®, and Bextra®),[4] may actually cause certain features of osteoarthritis to progress faster.[5,6,7] In addition, these new drugs can have other poten-tially serious side effects (see chapter 7 for more on this).

So, after years of masking your pain with drugs while your disease becomes progressively more severe, you may have to call in a surgeon to replace your hips or knees with artificial ones. Even with the new joint, however, you don't have as much function as you did before your arthritis developed. Surgery is painful, expensive, and not permanent—in ten years or so the replacement will probably begin to fail and the operation will probably have to be redone. And every time you have surgery, there's always the risk of dying or becoming permanently dis-abled from complications. But as the doctor said, there's nothing else to be done for osteoarthritis. Or is there?

A New Approach Emerges

Instead of simply dulling arthritis pain with drugs or performing expensive and potentially dangerous surgery, many doctors today are actually *curing* the symptoms of osteoarthritis. How? With three safe, inexpensive, readily available dietary supplements: glucosamine, chon-droitin, and a newly available supplement called ASU. These three supplements can be purchased without a prescription in almost any drug store or health-food store in America. The facts about this revolu-tionary but simple approach to solving a widespread problem are amazing:

- Since they are substances we already consume, and also produce in very small quantities in our bodies, glucosamine and chondroitin have no known significant side effects. This amazing fact stands in stark contrast to painkillers such as the nonsteroidal anti-inflammatories and cortisone injections, which can wreak havoc on the body.
- ASU, made from highly purified and concentrated fractions of avocado and soybean oil, is also safe and extremely well-tolerated. It has been used in France as a mainstay treatment for osteoarthritis for a number of years, with excellent results. Like glucosamine/chondroitin, ASU is now known to be the third, disease-improving treatment for osteoarthritis.
- An extensive body of clinical research—decades' worth—proves that glucosamine/chondroitin and ASU work in both humans and animals.
- Although these safe and effective therapies have long been used by physicians in Europe and elsewhere, they have been largely overlooked by the American medical community. Fortunately, this is starting to change. *We are now on the brink of a revolutionary improvement in the treatment of osteoarthritis and a revolutionary change in the way people think about this disease.*

The problem and its solution can be neatly summed up: Millions of Americans suffer from osteoarthritis, a painful and debilitating disease. Millions more are developing osteoarthritis now but do not yet have any symptoms. Osteoarthritis, the number-one cause of chronic pain, is one of the most widespread diseases in Western society. Although most physicians consider it to be incurable, osteoarthritis can actually be stopped in its tracks by using glucosamine/chondroitin and ASU. (These amazing natural substances may also be effective against other musculoskeletal conditions.) This astonishing information is well known and widely accepted in many other countries across the globe. The original edition of *The Arthritis Cure* brought the good news about glucosamine and chondroitin to the United States in 1997 and over 60 countries thereafter. Since then, these supplements have been widely accepted by most physicians, but some others still aren't convinced. They're concerned about accepting medical advances that come from abroad.

After all, we have a wonderful medical system. If something is that good, shouldn't American doctors have thought of it first? Shouldn't they at least know about it? And what about quality control and scientific studies? Aren't they less rigorous outside the United States? American doctors may not like to admit it, but physicians in other countries are often ahead of us in many areas of medicine. The first heart transplant was performed in South Africa; the first "test tube" baby was born in England; France was a forerunner in the development of the AIDS drug AZT. Angioplasty (using a balloon to open clogged arteries) and coronary stents (devices used to hold the artery open after an angioplasty) originated in Europe and are more advanced there than they are in the United States. Medications in Europe are rigorously tested and regulated, just as they are here. In fact, many drugs widely used in the United States and two-thirds of drugs overall, such as omeprazole (Prilosec®), were developed overseas.

We certainly have a good medical system, but it has traditionally been slow to accept new therapies or ideas. This is partially due to the federal Food and Drug Administration's decidedly unfriendly attitude toward the use of vitamins and other supplements for anything other than assuring that you meet your recommended daily nutritional requirements. And it's partially due to a relative lack of solid research into alternatives here in the United States. Indeed, a fair amount of the best scientific research on alternative approaches has been conducted in Germany and other European countries. The studies haven't all been translated into English, so they're not widely read by physicians here in the United States. Still, it's quite surprising that treatments used so successfully overseas for such a widespread and debilitating ailment have gone largely unnoticed in this country. Fortunately, that has started to change.

What Is Osteoarthritis?

The literal Greek translation of the word osteoarthritis is *osteo* (of the bone), *arthro* (joint), and *itis* (inflammation). But "bone/joint inflammation" may not be the most accurate description of osteoarthritis, since joint *pain* rather than inflammation is its most important characteristic. Indeed, while inflammation is a characteristic of many forms of arthritis, it is *not* found in most cases of osteoarthritis. This may be why some physicians feel that we should call the problem arthrosis, which means "degenerative joint disease."

Osteoarthritis is just one of many forms of joint disease. It is, however, the most common form of arthritis, affecting the articular cartilage, the smooth, glistening, bluish-white substance attached to ends of the bones. (Have you ever looked at or touched the end of a chicken drumstick? That's articular cartilage.) In fact, articular cartilage is one of the smoothest substances known. In addition to the articular cartilage, osteoarthritis, called OA for short, affects several other areas in and around the joints. These include:

- the subchondral bone (the ends of the bones, where the cartilage is attached)
- the capsules that surround the joints
- the muscles adjacent to the joint

The pain of osteoarthritis comes not just from the damaged articular cartilage but from the rest of the joint and the area around it. That's why exercise to strengthen the muscles supporting the joint is a part of the arthritis cure (see chapter 8 for more about this).

Cartilage: The Focal Point of Osteoarthritis

Osteoarthritis begins in the cartilage, the rubbery, gel-like tissue found at the ends of bones. About 65 to 80 percent water, cartilage is designed to do two things: reduce the friction caused by one bone rubbing against another, and blunt the constant trauma inflicted on bones during everyday life.

Think of healthy cartilage as being something like a sponge between the hard ends of the bones. This spongy material soaks up liquid (specifically, synovial fluid, the fluid found naturally in your joints) when the joint is at rest. When you move the joint and put pressure on it, the liquid is squeezed out again. For example, every time you take a step, your leg supports the pressure of your body weight. With each step, the cartilage in your knee joint is squeezed, forcing much of the synovial fluid out of it. But then when you pick up your foot to take another step, the fluid rushes back into the cartilage. The fluid "squishes" in and out as the cartilage responds to the constantly changing force exerted on the joint. Unlike a sponge, however, healthy cartilage does not flatten so easily. Filled with negatively charged *chondroitin* molecules that repel one another, increasing weight on the cartilage causes an increase in the repelling force. This is the same thing

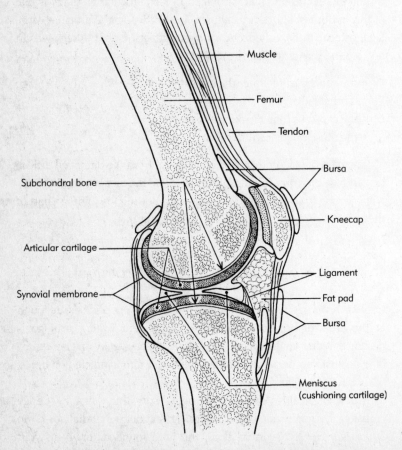

Fig. 1.1. Schematic of joint showing components.

that happens when you try to push two magnets together that are trying to repel each other. It gets harder and harder to keep the magnets together the closer they are in proximity to each other.

Over time, unfortunately, osteoarthritis can cause the loss of the chondroitin molecules and other cartilage components, eroding this protective buffer between the bones. As you'll learn in chapter 2, the problem has been growing in the cartilage matrix, the "birthplace" of cartilage, long before any symptoms are felt. As the disease progresses, the cartilage begins to soften and crack. The magnetic repelling effect is diminished and the cartilage cells die. In advanced cases, bone spurs (osteophytes), abnormal bone hardening (sclerosis or eburnation), and fluid-filled pockets in the bone (subchondral cysts) can form. And, of course, the more the cartilage wears away, the more the bones rub together, creating greater amounts of pain, bone deformities, and eventually inflammation. In severe cases the cartilage may disappear altogether, leaving the bone ends completely exposed in some places.

You can easily see cartilage damage and erosion by looking at an X ray of an osteoarthritic joint. The joint is narrowed and uneven—it's no longer held wide apart with the even contours of healthy cartilage. In fact, if you could actually look inside an arthritic joint, you'd immediately notice two things that distinguish it from a healthy one: First, the cartilage is breaking down, revealing an uneven, pitted surface that might even have holes in it. Second, new cartilage and new bone is being laid down by the body in an attempt to compensate for what has been lost. Unfortunately, this new cartilage and bone tissue can't completely replace what has been lost, and it is inferior to the original, healthy tissue.

Pain, Stiffness, and Other Forms of Misery

After many months or years of unnoticed damage to the cartilage, symptoms besides loss of flexibility or range-of-motion of the joints may become apparent. The major symptoms of osteoarthritis are pain, stiffness, crackling, and enlargement and deformities of the afflicted joint or joints, with inflammation possible in the advanced stages.

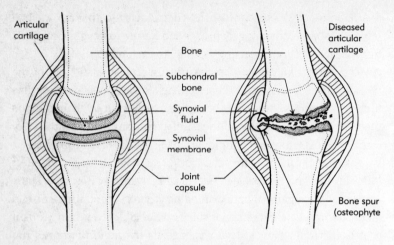

Fig. 1.2. A normal vs. osteoarthritic joint.

Pain.   The hallmark of osteoarthritis is pain described by patients as anything from a mild to moderately dull aching to a deep and throbbing pain. It usually begins as a minor ache that appears only after the joint has been used; the pain often disappears with rest. Cartilage itself doesn't have any nerve endings, so you don't feel the loss of cartilage until the osteoarthritis is actually fairly advanced and portions of the bone are exposed. Bone *does* have nerve endings—lots of them—and so do all of the major structures around a joint. The pain of OA comes from a variety of sources, including the places where muscles, ligaments, and tendons attach to the bones of the joint, the bone covering, the bone cavity, and inflammation around the joint capsule. As the disease progresses, a sharp pain may strike as soon as the joint is moved or used even a little. Eventually the joint aches even when it's in a resting position, unused and unpressured. In severe cases, osteoarthritic pain can disrupt sleep, making life even more miserable.

Stiffness.   Osteoarthritic joints are often stiff, especially for the first couple of minutes in the morning. They may also "lock up" after long periods of inactivity, such as sitting in a car or a movie theater. Early in the disease process, the stiffness lasts only briefly and can easily be "worked out" when you start to move again. But as the disease worsens, a permanent loss of range of motion occurs, one that doesn't improve even with warmup exercises and continual motion. Stiffness from OA isn't always associated with pain. In fact, some people develop severe stiffness without any pain. Don't assume you don't have OA just because you don't have pain. If you've noticed that you've become a little stiff and have lost some range of motion—you find it harder to bend down to pick something up off the floor, for instance—osteoarthritis could be the cause.

Joint crackling. Also known as crepitus, the crackling sound and crunching feeling coming from the affected joint(s) (most often a knee and less commonly a hip) usually indicates cartilage that is roughened or fragmented (normal, smooth cartilage is silent). As frightening as it sounds, crepitus is usually painless until some of the underlying bone is exposed or if cartilage fragments lead to inflammation in the joint. The sound may be more pronounced in advanced stages of osteo-arthritis. It may be caused by the joints rubbing together during regular use, or when the joint is passively manipulated during a medical examination. Most often striking the knees, the "creaking" sound can sometimes be heard all the way across a room!

Deformity and joint enlargement/inflammation. As the carti-lage degenerates, its shock absorption properties are decreased. The body tries to compensate for this and keep the bones from getting small microfractures by adding bone to help strengthen the joint. This leads to an enlargment of the bone and sometimes bone spurs. Bone spurs, also called osteophytes, can tug on the joint capsule or the cov-ering of the bone (called the periosteum), leading to further pain and inflammation. When this phenomenon occurs in the finger joints, it's usually from one of two conditions: Heberden's nodes or Bouchard's nodes. Heberden's nodes can disfigure the joints of the fingers closest to the fingertips, while Bouchard's nodes can cause enlargement of the middle joints of the fingers. (Heberden's nodes and Bouchard's nodes are more prevalent among women. They are thought to be an inherited form of osteoarthritis, since they often occur in members of the same family.)

Other symptoms.   OA may also cause bone cysts, gross bony overgrowth, bowed legs, and knock knees. Excess synovial fluid in the joint can also be a problem. In some cases, a doctor may have to take out as much as 100 milliliters of fluid (about four ounces) from a single osteoarthritic joint.

Although osteoarthritis can strike any joint, its "favorite" targets are the fingers, weight-bearing joints such as the knees and hips, the neck, lower back, and some joints in the feet. Most of the disability is caused by hip and knee OA, however, since this affects your ability to walk and exercise more than the other areas.

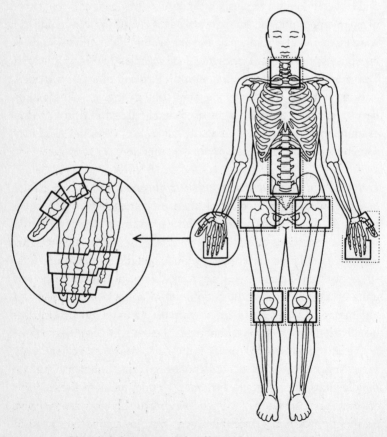

Fig. 1.3. Joints commonly affected by osteoarthritis.

Osteoarthritis can appear in one or more joints anywhere in the body, in no particular order, but it usually does not strike symmetrically (that is, not in *both* hips or *both* knees, at least not at first). When someone first develops hip or knee OA, he or she often favors the affected area and places more stress on the opposite side, causing the cartilage there to break down more quickly. OA can then develop in the opposite joint as well. OA doesn't travel like a rash, as some people believe; the adjacent or opposite joints become affected because of the extra load they have to bear to compensate for favoring the area affected first.

Primary Versus Secondary Osteoarthritis

Osteoarthritis appears in two general forms: primary and secondary.

Primary osteoarthritis, the more common form, is a slow and progressive condition that usually strikes after the age of 45, affecting mostly the weight-bearing joints of the knees and hips, as well as the lower back, neck, large toe joint, and fingers. Primary osteoarthritis usually develops in one of two ways: when excessive loads are placed on normal joint tissues (cartilage and subchondral bone), or when a reasonable load is applied on inferior joint tissues. The exact cause of primary osteoarthritis has not yet been determined, although family history and obesity are known risk factors.

The famous Framingham Heart Study, which began in 1948 and is still continuing, was primarily designed to identify the causes of heart disease in a large group of people who were followed over the course of decades. As part of the Framingham study, researchers also looked into the origins of osteoarthritis. What they found was a conclusive link between this disease and obesity. The study showed that obese people are more likely to develop osteoarthritis than are their slim counterparts.[8] And no wonder! The knees and hips, which are the primary weight-bearing joints of the body, handle loads anywhere from 2.5 to 10 times a person's body weight. This means that if you weigh 200 pounds, some of your joints may be handling as much as a ton of pressure as you walk, run, squat or otherwise use them. Clearly, the load on your joints can become incredibly difficult to bear as your body weight increases. Researchers have found that middle-aged women can greatly reduce their risk of developing osteoarthritis simply by losing weight. (You'll learn more about this crucial subject in chapter 9.)

Heredity also appears to play a role in the development of primary osteoarthritis. Researchers have long known that osteoarthritis tends to run in families, which suggests a strong genetic component. For instance, a study in 2000 showed that if you have severe OA in the hip, there's a very good chance that one or more of your siblings will have the same problem. Numerous studies have suggested a number of different genes as the culprits, but so far there's no one gene that can be identified as *the* arthritis gene.[9]

Secondary osteoarthritis is quite different from the primary form. Secondary simply means that the osteoarthritis appears as the result of some other known condition. As we learn more about arthritis, some patients who were classified as primary OA sufferers are found to have a known cause for their disease and are subsequently reclassified. In the future, we may actually classify OA as a number of separate conditions, each with specific features and properties.

Secondary osteoarthritis often appears before the age of 45 and has clearly defined causes: trauma or injury, joint laxity (a loose or "trick" knee, for example), joint infection, metabolic imbalances (gout or calcium deposits, iron overload, thyroid diseases, or chronic use of certain medications), or even just joint surgery.

Trauma appears to be the main culprit in secondary osteoarthritis, especially in younger people. The trauma can be *acute* (such as a sudden, serious injury) or *chronic* (recurring over time). Chronic trauma causes cumulative damage to the joint, one little "ouch" after another. The individual "ouches" may not be particularly severe, but added together over long periods of time, they can cause the joint tissues to fail. You'll often see chronic trauma in a joint that's unstable or "loose" because a supporting ligament was torn sometime in the past.

Repetitive impact loading is another form of chronic trauma. Repetitive impact loading involves repeated motions that traumatize the joint. A baseball pitcher throwing a ball hundreds of thousands of times, a pneumatic drill operator absorbing the vibrations of his drill in his shoulders for years, and a ballerina going from a flat foot to standing on her toes can all suffer from repetitive impact loading. Given time, these repeated motions can damage the cartilage and subchondral bone and cause secondary osteoarthritis. Repetitive impact loading is a major cause of secondary osteoarthritis, especially in joints already suffering from abnormal alignment or that are used in ways that they aren't meant to be.

Not all high-stress activities damage the joints. For example, the graceful divers of Acapulco who daily plunge from heights of more than 100 feet do not suffer from osteoarthritis of the spine. Researchers have no explanation for the divers' apparent immunity. Most of us aren't like these divers, however, and the wear and tear of high-stress activities over time often lead to osteoarthritis.

Your osteoarthritis may also be caused by poor bone alignment, joints that are not formed "quite right," or by something as simple as the way you walk. In addition to a careful biomechanical examination, using today's advanced computer technology and high-speed video cameras, doctors can infer what might be happening inside your joints. They can find out how well your joints function under pressure, whether there are biological abnormalities, if your gait or stride length is contributing to your osteoarthritis, and how walking or running on different surfaces affects your joints. If what's "bugging" your joints is simply that they're being stressed in an abnormal way, your doctor and physical therapist can devise special ways of "unloading" them, removing excessive pressure. Techniques for taking a load off your joints include:[10]

CHANGING YOUR BODY INTERNALLY
- brief periods of rest
- losing weight, if necessary
- manipulating tight structures (muscles, tendons, connective tissues, or joint capsules) that lead to strain on adjacent areas
- exercises designed to help spread the forces of everyday activity to many joints, which helps protect the arthritic joint
- strengthening muscles and other structures around the joint

CHANGING YOUR EXTERNAL ENVIRONMENT
- using a cane in the hand on the side opposite the affected lower extremity joint
- using soft neck collars, shoulder slings, splints on the wrists or fingers, and back corsets for brief periods of acute pain
- changing your chair, bed, flooring or exercise conditions (for example, walking on dirt or grass instead of cement or asphalt, or standing on carpet, rubber, or wood)
- wearing athletic or soft-soled shoes, and replacing them frequently
- using special shock-absorbing shoes called Z-coiLs

Who Is Affected by Osteoarthritis?

Arthritis afflicts countless millions of people worldwide, including nearly 70 million Americans, or one in three adults. Osteoarthritis, the most common form, is more prevalent than all other forms combined. It strikes all animals with bony skeletons, including birds, amphibians, and reptiles—even underwater mammals such as whales and porpoises.[11] And it seems as if osteoarthritis has plagued just about anything with bones since the beginning of time. The famous Roman baths were originally used to ease the pain of arthritic joints. Archaeologists have found evidence of osteoarthritis in Egyptian mummies, and paleontologists have discovered it in the skeletons of early humans dating back half a million years. In fact, the dinosaurs had it 200 million years ago.

Between 33 and 66 percent of any given group of people is afflicted with osteoarthritis. The statistics aren't exact, but it's fair to say that about 2 percent of those under the age of 45, 30 percent of those between 45 and 64, and 63 to 85 percent of those over the age of 65 suffer from osteoarthritis.[12] The true numbers may actually be higher, for many people with osteoarthritis have not yet developed symptoms. Among osteoarthritis victims under age 45, secondary osteoarthritis is more common, while primary osteoarthritis is rare.

Men are more likely to suffer from osteoarthritis than are women up to the age of 45, perhaps because males tend to engage in more strenuous physical activities and are more likely to suffer serious joint injuries.

From age 45 to 55, however, men and women begin to have an equal chance of suffering, while women are more likely victims after the age of 55. Not only is osteoarthritis more frequent in women age 55 or older, but the symptoms are also more severe. Millions of women of all ages have osteoarthritis and are affected about twice as often as men.

Osteoarthritis patterns vary according to ethnic background. For example, osteoarthritis of the hips is rarely seen in Japan and Saudi Arabia but is quite common in the United States.

Osteoarthritis Is Not Rheumatoid Arthritis

Osteoarthritis and rheumatoid arthritis are often confused because their names are similar and they both afflict the joints. But they are very different diseases. Rheumatoid arthritis is an autoimmune disorder that can lead to weakness, fatigue, fever, anemia, and other problems, including inflamed joints. (An autoimmune disorder is one in which the body attacks its own tissues, as if they were foreign invaders.) Rheumatoid arthritis tends to strike symmetrically, which means that it hits both sides of the body at once (both wrists, both hands, and so on). Some two and a half million people in the United States have rheumatoid arthritis.[13] The chart below shows some of the major distinctions between osteoarthritis and the far less common rheumatoid arthritis:

Osteoarthritis	Rheumatoid Arthritis
Usually begins after age 40.	Initially strikes between the ages of 25 and 50.
Develops gradually over several years.	Often comes and goes without warning.
Usually begins in joints on one side of the body.	Usually attacks joints on both sides of the body simultaneously (e.g., both hands).
Redness, warmth, and swelling (inflammation) of joints is unusual.	Redness, warmth, and swelling (inflammation) of joints is universal.

Osteoarthritis	Rheumatoid Arthritis
Primarily affects joints of the hands, hips, feet, and spine. Only occasionally attacks the knuckles, wrists, elbows, or shoulders.	Affects many or most joints, knees, including the knuckles, wrists, elbows, and shoulders.
Doesn't cause an overall feeling of sickness.	Often causes an overall feeling of sickness and fatigue, as well as weight loss and fever.

Diagnosing the Joint Malady

Before making a diagnosis of osteoarthritis, a good doctor will carefully note your complaints, review your medical history, and examine you from head to toe. During the examination he or she will look for several distinct signs, such as limited range of motion in the joints, tenderness to touch (palpation), pain upon bending and flexing your joint (passive motion), and joint crackling and grinding (crepitus).

Limited range of motion in the joints. At first, the inability to move a joint as well as before may be subtle and hard to measure, but with time the limitation of movement becomes obvious. If the osteoarthritis is in the hand, for example, you may have difficulty opening a jar or grasping a ball. If it's in the knee, bending or extending the joint can become very uncomfortable. If your spine is affected, you may have trouble twisting or bending. And if the problem is severe enough, the weight-bearing joints of the hips and knees may not be well enough for you to do simple activities. Fine hand movements such as pinching are not usually affected by osteoarthritis.

Tenderness to touch. The joint may not feel tender at all in the early stages of the disease, but as OA progresses swelling can develop as the body produces more synovial fluid in the joint. The excess fluid puts pressure on the tissues surrounding the joint, which causes pain and tenderness to the touch. Bone spurs and inflamed tendon and ligament attachments can also be sensitive areas and may cause pain that seems to be outside the joint.

Pain with passive motion.   We don't normally know if we have pain upon passive motion because our movement is almost always active. It's usually only when a doctor moves our arms and legs about that we experience passive movement. Many times, however, we'll feel pain and a crunching or creaking of the bones when the doctor manually bends and flexes our afflicted joints. In addition to checking for these physical signs of osteoarthritis, the doctor will request a simple X ray to confirm the diagnosis. Osteoarthritis shows up on an X ray first by changes in the bone just beneath the cartilage. Narrowing of the joint spaces is often seen as well. In advanced cases, bones spurs, abnormal denseness, abnormal joint alignment, and pockets of fluid in the bone (bone cysts) may also be apparent. Osteophytes, or bone spurs, which can be seen on an X ray, are a sign that the bone is trying to repair itself in order to support the load on an affected joint.

More sophisticated imaging techniques, such as arthrography, CT (computerized tomography) scans, and MRI (magnetic resonance imaging), may also be used to help assess the extent of cartilage damage, but these are not yet the standard and your health insurance may not pay for these tests if they are done solely to diagnosis osteoarthritis. MRI scanning is rapidly becoming the most sensitive (and earliest indicator) of the radiographic techniques to detect OA. Sometimes fluid from the joint will be removed for analysis to differentiate OA from gout, infection, or other causes of swelling. A good doctor will spend some time exploring secondary causes of OA so the root of the problem may be uncovered before treatment begins. A more comprehensive list of these causes is available at www.drtheo.com.

What Does Not *Cause Osteoarthritis?*

Despite plenty of evidence to the contrary, three common misconceptions about osteoarthritis persist: that it is a normal part of the aging process, that it is simply a "wear and tear" disease, and that it cannot be halted or reversed. Nothing could be further from the truth! Osteoarthritis is *not* inevitable—there are things you can do now to prevent or delay the onset of OA. We used to believe that the joint deterioration found with aging was the same kind of deterioration seen in those with osteoarthritis. Now we know that there are striking differences between joints and cartilage that are affected by osteoarthritis and those that have simply aged normally. These differences are described in the chart below.

Aged Joints	Osteoarthritic Joints
Deterioration occurs on *non*-weight-bearing cartilage surfaces.	Deterioration occurs on weight-bearing cartilage surfaces.
Minimal physical and chemical change in the cartilage matrix.	Significant physical, chemical, and degradative changes in the cartilage matrix
No increase in tissue volume.	Increase in tissue volume.
No change in the liquid content of the cartilage.	Early and dramatic increase in the liquid content of cartilage. (This may be the first physical change.)
Pigment in cartilage.	No pigment in cartilage.
No bone sclerosis or eburnation (excess bone denseness or overgrowth).	Sclerosis and eburnation.
No obvious bone changes.	Bone changes, including abnormal new bone formation (osteophytes).

While it is true that osteoarthritis occurs more frequently and severely in older persons, this is due to prolonged exposure to the everyday traumas and repetitive motions that occur throughout a lifetime and a decrease in the ability for minor self-repair. While osteoarthritis may occur more often and with more severity as we age, it is not *caused* by the aging process.

Primary osteoarthritis is *not* caused by wear and tear on the body due to strenuous activity or exercise. Recent scientific studies have conclusively proven that regular exercise does not predispose us to osteoarthritis. In fact, the opposite is true: vigorous exercise actually *increases* the functional status of those with osteoarthritis.[14] Secondary arthritis due to injuries or repetitive impact loading may be caused by use and abuse of a joint, but normal amounts of exercise actually help to *prevent* primary arthritis and can play a major role in treating the disease.

We *can* relieve the pain and disability of osteoarthritis. Most doctors in the United States shrug their shoulders and accept the "inevitable" when treating patients with osteoarthritis, prescribing nothing more than painkillers. But advances in the understanding of cartilage and years of experience with numerous patients have shown that it is definitely possible to slow, halt, or prevent the degeneration of cartilage that is characteristic of osteoarthritis. Specifically, there is strong evidence suggesting that restoring the normal balance to the cartilage matrix can have a positive impact on the course and outcome of the disease.[15]

The traditionally minded American medical establishment has been slowly adapting to the dramatic changes in the field of osteoarthritis. The growing body of evidence is beginning to force doctors to reevaluate their thinking and to open their minds to the promise of the treatment program described in *The Arthritis Cure.* Today more and more physicians suggest that their patients with OA use glucosamine/chondroitin; in the future, they will also suggest using ASU. Doctors are slowly beginning to realize that osteoarthritis is *not* inevitable, and that it may even be cured.

There Is *Hope*

Osteoarthritis is a very common affliction that most doctors in the United States think is both inevitable and incurable. Fortunately, they are wrong! The Arthritis Cure has helped to relieve the pain of osteoarthritis and slow the disease for many people around the world, allowing them to once again enjoy normal and productive lives.

2

WHEN JOINTS GO BAD

How does a joint work?

What is cartilage made of?

What happens when cartilage degenerates?

Can damaged cartilage be healed without using possibly dangerous medicines or surgery?

Shoulders, knees, elbows, hips, fingers, and more—the human body has 143 different joints, parts of which act as the hinges, levers, and shock absorbers that allow us to stand, walk, run, kneel, jump, dance, climb, sit, grasp, push, pull, shake hands, scratch our heads, eat, and otherwise perform the thousands of motions that get us through the day. Whether it's a large knee joint or a little toe joint, each is a complex unit that makes movement possible. These mechanical marvels hold bones close enough together to allow coordinated movement, while ensuring that they slide gently over each other, never sticking or grinding. Joints work so well that most people are completely unaware of them until something goes wrong.

Three Types of Joints

All of the joints in the human body fall into one of three categories: fixed, slightly moveable, or highly mobile. The differences in our joints allow us to achieve the perfect balance between stability and movement.

Fixed joints join together bones that have very little, if any, movement against each other, such as the suture joints that connect the bony plates that form the skull. Arthritis is not a problem in these stationary joints, which are called synarthrodial (sin-ar-THROW-dee-all) joints.

Slightly moveable joints bring together bones that can move a little bit with respect to each other, such as the sacroiliac joints, which connect the lowest part of the spine with the pelvis (thus connecting the upper and lower body). Called amphiarthrodial (am-fee-ar-THROW-dee-all) joints, they only occasionally succumb to osteoarthritis.

It's the highly mobile joints that are the chief targets of osteoarthritis. Also called diarthrodial (die-ar-THROW-dee-all) or synovial (si-NO-vee-all) joints, they come in many different forms. The elbows, for example, are hinge joints that allow the lower arms to swing up to meet the upper arms, much as a door swings open and closed. The ball-and-socket joints that connect the upper leg bones to the pelvis allow for a much wider range of motion than the hinge joints. You can move your legs forward and backward, to the left and to the right, or even around in a semicircular manner. Then there are saddle joints that bring together the bones at the base of the thumbs, gliding joints in the hand, carpal bones in the wrist, and more.

Highly mobile joints come in many different sizes and shapes, though they all have similar purposes and structures. They are designed to hold bones very close together while still allowing them to move smoothly against each other. Their structure, although complex, is much the same, whether they are hinge, ball-and-socket, saddle, or any other type of highly mobile joint. All joints have the same basic parts:

- the joint capsule, a tough membrane or "sack" that encloses the joint and connects one bone to another, holding them firmly in place
- the synovial (inner) lining of the joint capsule, which secretes *synovial fluid* to lubricate as well as to nourish the cartilage
- articular cartilage, the tough, rubbery substance that caps the ends of the bones and absorbs shock, while providing a slick surface so that the bone ends can easily glide across each other during movement

- ligaments, bands of tough, fibrous tissue that attach bones to bones and help provide stability within the joint
- tendons, bands of tough, fibrous tissue that attach muscles to bones, allow for movement, and act as secondary joint stabilizers
- muscles, tissues that contract to provide the force for movement and are critical for absorbing shock from around a joint
- bursae, small, fluid-filled sacs positioned at strategic points in and around joints to cushion ligaments and tendons, protecting them against friction and wear and tear

Now that you understand the basic elements of a joint, let's look more closely at the part that's most affected by osteoarthritis: the articular cartilage.

A Closer Look at Articular Cartilage

There are many types of cartilage, performing many different functions in the body, but when it comes to OA, we're primarily concerned with the articular cartilage, the cartilage found in the joints. Since this is the substance that must be present and healthy for smooth, pain-free movement in the joints, it's worth taking the time to examine it in greater detail.

To get an idea of what cartilage does, imagine rubbing together two perfectly flat, smooth, slightly wet ice cubes. They glide across each other quickly and easily, never catching or slowing. Now imagine a surface that's five to eight times more slippery than ice. That's your articular cartilage, the material that makes it possible for the ends of your bones to slide smoothly and easily across each other. In fact, no man-made substance can compare to the low-friction and shock-absorbing properties of healthy cartilage.

Like much of the body, cartilage is a watery substance—in fact, it's 65 to 80 percent water. The rest of it is made up of *collagen, cartilage cells (chondrocytes),* and *proteoglycans,* the substances that give cartilage its amazing properties of resilience and shock absorption. Together, water, collagen, and proteoglycans form the *cartilage matrix,* the "birthplace" of cartilage.

Collagen, proteins known for their versatility, is found in many different parts of the body, taking different forms to fulfill various functions. In fact, the fourteen varieties of collagen make up about half the protein in your body. Collagen is formed into strong ropes to make tendons, thin sheets to form skin, clear membranes to make corneas, and strong, weight-bearing structures that we call bones. A very specific form of collagen, type II, is a vital part of joint cartilage, providing it with elasticity and the ability to absorb shock. It also creates a framework to hold the proteoglycans in place.[1] In a sense, collagen is the "glue" that holds the cartilage matrix together.

Proteoglycans are huge molecules made up of protein and sugars. Looking a little like round bottle brushes or Christmas trees, proteoglycans are woven around and through the collagen fibers, forming a dense netting inside the cartilage. The proteoglycans make cartilage resilient so that it can stretch and then bounce back when we move.[2] The amazing proteoglycans also trap water. Imagine that you're holding a sponge under water. When you squeeze that sponge, water squirts out, only to rush back in as soon as you relax your grip. Thanks to the thirsty and resilient proteoglycans, your cartilage acts like that sponge, rapidly absorbing water in the form of synovial fluid when the pressure is off the joint, then squeezing it out again when the pressure is on. This allows cartilage to respond to our movements and absorb shock without cracking under the strain.

In addition to the collagen and proteoglycans, there are also special cells called *chondrocytes* sprinkled throughout the cartilage matrix. Chondrocytes are miniature factories that produce new collagen and proteoglycan molecules, always making sure that there are enough of these vital substances. But since everything in our bodies eventually ages and weakens, the chondrocytes also release enzymes to "chew up" and dispose of the aging collagen and proteoglycan molecules that have passed their prime.

When Physical Stress Damages Cartilage

These four elements of healthy cartilage—collagen, proteoglycans, chondrocytes, and water—work together to ensure smooth, pain-free movement. Unfortunately, several things can disrupt the careful teamwork, causing disease and painful distress. We don't know exactly what causes primary osteoarthritis, but we do know that secondary osteoarthritis is often caused by trauma. The trauma may be sudden and severe, such as a blow to the hip while playing football. Or perhaps the trauma is slow and gradual, the built-up effect of hundreds or thousands of tiny injuries. Obesity can also damage joints by forcing them to bear too much weight or perhaps by causing hormonal changes not yet identified.

Sometimes, joints become damaged simply because a person has inherited (or developed) a body that "wears" in an unfortunate manner. We do know that above a certain threshold, physical impact can cause normal cartilage cells to turn into "osteoarthritic" cells. The cartilage cells become enlarged and very active in both producing but mostly destroying cartilage.

Some recent research suggests that a precise mechanism involving a small fragment of collagen can trigger this transformation. It also appears that once the change takes place, it's difficult to turn off.[3]

Whatever the reason for the trigger in secondary OA, when the trauma occurs, the once-healthy cartilage begins to break down.

The surface of the damaged cartilage may become ragged and pockmarked. Eventually it may wear through completely, leaving holes that make it look like a moth-eaten sweater. Without healthy and whole cartilage to cushion them, the bones may begin to rub against each other, causing severe pain. The lack of cushioning may also make small fractures develop in the cartilage. Your body usually responds to this by producing more cartilage to plug the cracks, but the replacement cartilage is often inferior in quality, unable to cushion the bone ends against the forces of impact. As a result, the ends of those bones change, losing some of their ability to "bend" under stress and act as shock absorbers. Your body may then overproduce bone material for the bone ends in an attempt to correct the problem, but that only makes things worse by causing bumpy surfaces in the joint, enlargement of the joint, and bone spurs.

Whether it's the cartilage or the bone that's damaged, the result is trouble. Damaged, uneven cartilage is like a scraggly old carpet, and an overgrown bone is like a floor littered with sharp rocks. In either case, the joint no longer has smooth contours, so fluid, pain-free movement is impossible.

As the joint degenerates, the joint lining (synovium) often becomes inflamed. The synovium has many nerve endings and pain receptors, so inflammation invariably sends pain messages rocketing off to the brain. The synovium tries to solve the problem by producing more and more synovial fluid, the slick, watery substance that lubricates and nourishes the cartilage. This sounds like a good idea, but the resulting fluid isn't of the same quality as normal. The synovial fluid can sometimes end up flooding the joint space, causing swelling, limited range of motion, and perhaps even more pain. The synovium itself may also swell up and exude a puslike material.

That's what's happening inside the ailing joint. But all you're aware of is that your knee really hurts, it's swollen, it's hard to bend, and you don't want to put weight on it. And all this began with some type of triggering event.

Theories for the Primary Form of Osteoarthritis

Why do we even develop osteoarthritis? What good is it to have a built-in mechanism that causes cartilage to degenerate? Researchers don't know for sure, but one possibility is that your joints need some way to repair themselves, but they can't use the same type of repair system as most other parts of the body. Normally, when a tissue is injured, it bleeds, as when you cut your finger. Bleeding leads to a clot and then scar formation. This is all right for the skin or even muscles, but not for the joints. Joints need to be free of scar tissue that could limit movement. Also, scar tissue is not a good shock absorber and would easily break down from the force placed on the joint when it moves or bears weight.

The joints are a relatively closed system. A waterproof, fibrous capsule surrounds them, and there are no blood vessels in cartilage to carry nutrients into and waste products out of the joints. The transfer of nutrients occurs through an intermediary—blood vessels in the joint capsule exchange nutrients and waste with the joint (synovial) fluid.

If there were blood vessels in the cartilage, even a slight injury could cause bleeding. Blood in the joint could form a clot and eventually lead to a scar, which could quickly reduce the function of the joint by decreasing its range of motion and altering the way the joint absorbs shock. This isn't a good way to make repairs to a joint. We know this because severe joint injuries, such as a rupture of the ligaments within the joint or a joint dislocation, can cause bleeding, swelling, and a rapid decrease in joint function.

Instead, your body uses a system of chemical checks and balances to handle the many small, routine joint injuries that cause cartilage to tear or break off small fragments. A natural process of cartilage building and breakdown allows joints to degrade any loose fragments that might affect the their function. Without this ability to break down cartilage, some of these fragments might act as a doorstop and jam the motion of the joint.

Degrading the cartilage fragments is your body's only way to flush them out of the joint. (Orthopedic surgeons weren't around until recently.) One of the ways the fragments can be degraded is for the cartilage cells (chondrocytes) to sense joint damage and then start to produce chemicals (enzymes or cytokines) that have the ability to break down cartilage. Chondrocytes are normally very quiet in healthy cartilage—they don't have to produce many new cartilage molecules. After trauma, however, chondrocytes swing into action and become enlarged (hypertrophied) and very active. Once this process starts, however, it's not easy to stop. The chondrocytes can continue to degrade cartilage—even healthy cartilage that would have been fine if it was left alone. In time, this can lead to the gradual but steady breakdown of the cartilage that is the hallmark of osteoarthritis—a process in which the destruction of cartilage occurs faster than your body can repair it. Besides this imbalance in repair and degradation of cartilage, OA causes new cartilage production to differ from normal cartilage, as if it's being haphazardly created just to fill in the gaps. Increases in other kinds of collagen, such as types III, VI, and X appear. The new cartilage that forms isn't as sturdy as the original and it's more likely to break down later.

Up until the twentieth century, it didn't matter too much that the process of cartilage degradation seemed to be a one-way phenomenon—after destroying the damaged cartilage, the chondrocytes moved on to attack the healthy cartilage. That's because the life expectancy of the average person at the turn of the twentieth century was only about 46 years. Going back to earlier times, average life expectancy was even lower. With humans living such a short period of time, even if the osteoarthritis process started in someone who was in their teens or twenties, the slow degradation of cartilage might not even cause any symptoms of joint pain, much less leave them devoid of cartilage, before they died from another cause. The osteoarthritis from injury didn't matter, because most people didn't live long enough to experience the painful effects!

We know that physical stress is one cause of secondary osteoarthritis, but researchers have yet to determine the exact cause of primary osteoarthritis, Several theories have been developed to explain the genesis of this painful and puzzling problem.

Changes in the cartilage matrix.   The chondrocytes are responsible for maintaining the normal mix of collagen, proteoglycans, and water that make up the cartilage matrix. For unknown reasons, in OA the "recipe" gets scrambled and the proportions are altered. A possible cause of the faulty matrix is the accumulation of *advanced glycation end products* (AGEs) in the chondrocytes. Think of AGEs as waste products of metabolism that build up and interfere with the normal function of chondrocytes (and other cells, like "age spots" in the skin). The more AGEs that build up, the lower the ability of the chondrocytes to keep up their chores of maintaining the cartilage matrix. Think of it this way:

If you never took out the trash from your kitchen, you'd find it harder and harder to make dinner until one day, you wouldn't even be able to get into the kitchen at all!

The AGE theory of primary osteoarthritis is supported by increasing evidence and helps explain the greater frequency of OA in people with diabetes and the aged, two groups that have accelerated production of AGEs.

Changes in the subchondral bone.   Hardening of the subchondral bone that underlies the cartilage can reduce the bone's ability to deform under physical stress. This in turn can lead to increased pressure on the cartilage and perhaps chondrocytes, causing their early demise. Don't confuse this bone change with osteoporosis. There does not appear to be a significant relationship between osteoporosis (bone loss) and the development of (or protection from) osteoarthritis.

An enzyme or chemical signal in the cartilage may be out of control.   Chondrocytes produce collagen and proteoglycans, so the body may try to correct cartilage problems by manufacturing more chondrocytes, usually of the hypertrophied or hyperactive type. But these hypertrophied chondrocytes don't limit themselves to making cartilage-building materials—they also make enzymes that break down old collagen and proteoglycans. Extra chondrocytes mean more cartilage-building substances, but also more cartilage-busting enzymes. The net result may be the opposite of what was intended: More cartilage is destroyed than created. When a joint is flooded with these cartilage-chewing enzymes, the collagen fibers in the cartilage become smaller, and the dense netting that they provide becomes torn or pitted. The proteoglycans, which are normally held in place by the collagen, begin to drift off and decompose. Without enough proteoglycans around to attract and hold water, and repel the forces applied to the joint, the cartilage becomes more susceptible to cracking, fissuring, and wearing through completely. This can be seen under a microscope: Healthy proteoglycans look like thick, full Christmas trees, but damaged proteoglycans look like old, dead trees.

The cartilage-busting enzymes that the chondrocytes produce are normally kept in check by an equal number of cartilage-promoting enzymes. If the balance is off, or if too many of the cartilage-destroying enzymes are produced, the results can be disastrous. This imbalance in breakdown versus build-up of cartilage components is the hallmark of OA. It's what we try to restore through the supplements discussed in this book.

Bone disease.   A problem with the blood supply to the bone could weaken it, leading to small fractures and *osteonecrosis,* or "bone death." Alcoholism, infection, and acute trauma are among the possible culprits in this scenario.

Abnormal liver function.   Your liver is the source of many hormones, growth factors, and substances that aid cartilage and bone formation. If it's not functioning properly, bony overgrowth and cartilage destruction may be a result.

Can We Repair the Damage?

Whatever the cause may be, all OA sufferers seem to want to know the same things: Can the damage be repaired? Is there a way to make the cartilage surface slick and slippery again? Is it possible to repair and restore cartilage that was damaged long ago? Would fixing the cartilage cure the pain, inflammation, and bony overgrowth? And would that cure the arthritis?

Too often, people wait until very late in the course of the disease to get help. Usually by the time a person has symptoms of limited joint motion or persistent joint pain, the damage to the cartilage is severe, and the OA has been present for many years. Since most of the early changes in OA are chemical, or microscopic, it is difficult to diagnose OA in it earliest stages. There are no blood (or even joint fluid) tests universally accepted to show if a person has or does not have OA. X rays become positive only after years of disease, so in general X rays are not good at detecting early OA. MRI scans, which use a magnetic field and radio waves (but no X-ray radiation), can detect OA changes in cartilage much earlier and are becoming the new standard for diagnosing OA and for OA research. MRI scans are currently used mainly to look for torn cartilage or cartilage in the joints, or other joint problems such as death of the bone (osteonecrosis). Insurance companies will pay for the scans for these reasons because they figure a normal scan may deter the patient from having a costly surgery, but they usually don't pay for MRIs to diagnose osteoarthritis.

I believe the use of MRI scanning to detect OA will become more common and will be reimbursed, once insurance companies realize that by implementing the Arthritis Cure treatment program early on, they can save money on future drug and surgery costs, besides preventing years of suffering for their patients.

Nothing to date can reverse the changes to the bone or remove bone spurs, but intervening earlier in the disease has been shown to halt the cartilage destruction and reduce the other triggers leading to joint pain and loss of function. This is the basis of the "chondroprotective" theory of treating arthritis, an approach based on protecting cartilage cells. It is possible to stop the destruction of cartilage in osteoarthritis, to repair some of the lost cartilage, and to improve joint function. We *can* restore health and balance to the cartilage matrix *now*, without waiting for complex new surgeries or new medications to be perfected. We *can* often reduce or eliminate the pain and disability of osteoarthritis with a nine-step program that incorporates three safe, simple nutritional supplements: glucosamine, chondroitin, and ASU.

—3—

NEW HOPE FOR BEATING OSTEOARTHRITIS

*Can glucosamine/chondroitin truly modify the
course of osteoarthritis?*

What is glucosamine? How does it work?

What is chondroitin sulfate? How does it work?

Why are glucosamine/chondroitin used together?

*Do scientific studies support the use of
glucosamine/chondroitin?*

*Do other substances work with
glucosamine/chondroitin?*

What is the GAIT study?

*Why has it taken so long for
glucosamine/chondroitin to be used in the
United States?*

*Do I need a prescription to buy
glucosamine/chondroitin? Where can they
be purchased?*

Slim, well-toned 42-year-old Brett Jacobs was an exuberant amateur athlete. Although he worked hard at his job as vice president of advertising at a large toy firm, he still managed to jog several days a week, play basketball with the guys on Thursday nights, and pitch for the company softball team on the weekends.

And then one day his right knee began to hurt. It was a dull, aching pain on the inside of his knee that came and went for no apparent reason. At first it only struck while he was jogging or running up and down the basketball court, but soon he began to feel it while standing still, sitting at his desk, and finally even when he was sleeping. There was no pattern to the pain, except that it was steadily growing worse.

Fortunately, he had excellent medical insurance and was seen by the best orthopedists, neurologists, rheumatologists, internists, chiropractors, acupuncturists, and other specialists. But the exhaustive (although noninvasive) testing found absolutely nothing wrong with his knees—or with any other part of his body, for that matter. He took various pain medications, had physical therapy, and even got a steroid injection. Frustrated, he finally had arthroscopic surgery and was found to have some cartilage degeneration on the end of his thigh bone (femur). The surgeon felt that there was nothing that could be done surgically, especially since Brett's cartilage had not yet completely worn through. He essentially told Brett to "grin and bear it." But the pain grew continually worse, and within a year Brett had given up jogging, basketball, and baseball. He certainly wasn't grinning anymore.

Less than two years after the first mild pain appeared, Brett was forced to spend most of his day sitting in a chair, only standing and moving about when absolutely necessary. Luckily, his job allowed him to sit at a desk most of the day. But he missed his active life. When his friends would ask him if he'd ever be able to join them in sports again, he would sigh heavily and say: "No, I'm hanging up my running shoes. My old life as an active person is over, and now I'm the gold-medal champion sitter-downer. But the good news is that with all the aspirin I'm taking for my knee, there's no chance I'll ever have another headache."

Depressed, Brett had given up all hope of ever being able to walk without pain. Then he heard about glucosamine and chondroitin on a radio show about health and nutrition. They were only mentioned briefly, but Brett decided to give them a try. Two weeks after he started taking glucosamine/chondroitin, he said, "I stopped taking the aspirin, just to see what would happen. I was surprised to see that my knee didn't hurt much anymore. So I started standing up and walking around a little, just a little. I kept taking the glucosamine and chondroitin. A couple weeks after that I started pushing it, walking all the way around the block, just to see what would happen. It was great, no pain! I added a little more activity every week. One week I increased my walking to ten minutes a day, the next week to fifteen, the next to twenty. Then I added in riding the bicycle at the club for five minutes, the next week for ten minutes, and so on. Little by little I did more and more until I was actually jogging again. Only a mile at first, but I was actually doing it! Then I started adding in a little baseball, then a little basketball, then a little more, and a little more. Now I'm doing just about everything I used to do."

Six months after he started taking glucosamine/chondroitin, Brett was once again lacing on his jogging shoes, playing weekend softball, and shooting hoops with his friends. "I'm 90 percent back," he now says with a grin, "hoping to be 100 percent soon!"

Patients aren't the only ones raving about these two arthritis-busting nutritional supplements. Doctors in Europe and Asia have been successfully using glucosamine/chondroitin for years to treat osteoarthritis. In the United States, most physicians who are knowl-edgeable in the area of osteoarthritis are now recommending these supplements, often as first-line therapy before pain relievers or anti-inflammatory medications. Once doctors read the evidence, they can't avoid the fact that the supplements are sometimes more effective and far safer than the drugs they had been recommending. As one doctor told me, "According to our Hippocratic oath, we should do no harm. After reading a number of the studies, including head-to-head com-parisons with anti-inflammatory drugs, I have found it difficult from an ethical standpoint to *not* recommend glucosamine and chondroitin first, before the Tylenol, Celebrex, or Advil." As the message gets out further, it is only a matter of time before we see this type of attitude in the medical establishment as a whole.

Just Imagine

Healthy cartilage needs three things: water for lubrication and nour-ishment, proteoglycans to attract and hold the water, and collagen to keep the proteoglycans in place.

Imagine a dense netting made up of countless ropes woven together, some going up and down, others running from side to side to form a mesh. Healthy cartilage has a similar structure. Its "threads" are tough, ropy collagen, laid down at right angles to each other in a criss-cross pattern, many layers thick.

Proteoglycans anchor themselves securely in place in the spaces in the collagen "netting" by wrapping themselves over, under, around, and through the collagen threads. The proteoglycans are absolutely essential for healthy cartilage, for they attract and hold many times their weight in water, which lubricates, nourishes, and contributes to the cartilage's function. The water in the cartilage assists in the shock-absorbing properties, behaving much like the water in a waterbed if you tried to walk or jump on it. But if the cartilage is damaged, or if the cartilage-chewing enzymes go wild, the netting becomes weak and frays. As the netting loses its shape and unwinds, proteoglycans lose their grip and float away, only to be digested by enzymes that break them down. Without these water-attracting molecules in place, the cartilage loses its ability to absorb shock and the cartilage cells die, unable to keep up with the demand of producing more cartilage matrix or to get the nourishment they require. Without the cartilage cells, it is only a matter of time before the rest of the cartilage matrix starts to fray, fissure, and eventually wear down to the bone. Then, once the bone becomes exposed, the nerve endings become irritated, leading to the characteristic joint pain. Without the protective effect of the cartilage and the thick, nourishing joint fluid (called hyaluronan or hyaluronic acid) produced by the chondrocytes, the underlying bone is exposed to more and more pressure. In an effort to prevent the joint from suffering small fractures, the bone cells start to lay down more hard bone mineral. This leads to a hardening of the bone, growth of bone spurs and an increase in the size of the joint. In many cases, the bone spurs and bony overgrowths will stretch, pull, or pinch on some of the structures around the joint. Sometimes fragments of bone and cartilage break off, causing the joint to grind or even catch and lock. The result of all of this degeneration is the familiar signs and symptoms of advanced osteoarthritis: pain, inflammation, and swelling, along with "mechanical" symptoms of catching, locking, and loss of flexibility.

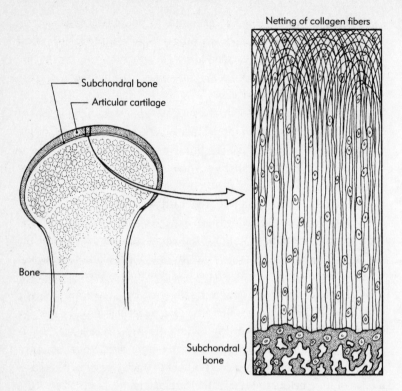

Fig. 3.1. Composition and structure of cartilage.

Building the "Water Holders"

How does glucosamine figure into healthy cartilage? Glucosamine is made up of glucose (the sugar your body burns for fuel) and an amino acid called glutamine. It is an important part of the mucopolysaccharides, which provide structure to the bone, cartilage, skin, nails, hair, and other body tissues. *Glucosamine* is a major building block of the water-loving proteoglycans. Specifically, glucosamine is needed to make *glycosaminoglycans* (GAGs), large, chainlike molecules that bind water in the cartilage matrix. Beside providing raw material for the synthesis of proteoglycans and other GAGs, glucosamine's mere presence acts as a stimulant to the cells that produce these products, the *chondrocytes*.[1] In fact, glucosamine is the key factor in determining how many proteoglycans are produced by the chondrocytes. If there is a lot of glucosamine present, then a lot of proteoglycans will be produced, and a lot of water will be held in its proper place. But if only a little glucosamine is available, fewer proteoglycans will be made, and less of the precious water will be attracted to the area. Glucosamine has also been shown to spur the chondrocytes to produce more collagen and proteoglycans, and it also normalizes cartilage metabolism, which helps to keep the cartilage from breaking down.[2]

Recent studies of glucosamine have shown us other ways in which glucosamine benefits the health of the cartilage and the joints. We now know that glucosamine also helps decrease the production of enzymes that break down the cartilage,[3] helps keep the cartilage cells adhering to the cartilage matrix,[4] and helps decrease the production of a signaling chemical called nitric oxide.[5] (Nitric oxide has been shown to lead to early cartilage cell death.) Finally, in one study, glucosamine actually inhibited the COX-2 enzyme,[6] which may explain why glucosamine can actually decrease inflammation and give some people symptomatic relief in a very short period of time (you'll learn more about this in chapter 7 on painkillers).

Because glucosamine "jump-starts" the production of these key elements of the cartilage matrix, and then protects them, *it can actually help the body to repair damaged or eroded cartilage*. In other words, glucosamine strengthens your body's natural repair mechanisms.

Many scientific studies have shown that besides stimulating the production of cartilage, glucosamine helps to reduce pain and improve joint function in those with osteoarthritis.[7,8] It doesn't seem to matter if the glucosamine is manufactured by your body or comes from a supplement. Supplemental glucosamine acts just like the glucosamine that we eat in very small quantities in our food and the glucosamine found naturally in our cartilage. Where it comes from isn't important. It just needs to be present. And glucosamine continues to work even after the treatment stops.

Forms of Glucosamine

In the United States, glucosamine supplements are available without a prescription in three forms—hydrochloride, N-acetyl, and sulfate. These other components are attached to the glucosamine base molecule to give it a stable structure so it can be used as a powder in supplements. You can't buy free glucosamine base alone, and you really wouldn't want to, because unattached glucosamine is unstable. It would quickly become inactive or want to bind to something else.

Regulated and sold as a drug in Europe, glucosamine sulfate is the form that is used in most research. About 75 percent of all clinical research on glucosamine has been performed with a stabilized form of glucosamine sulfate. Much of the basic science and animal research has been performed with glucosamine hydrochloride, so we know it is effective also. No clinical study to date has compared the effects of the hydrochloride form to the sulfate form of glucosamine. But equivalence has been shown in the lab. On the other hand, there is evidence to suggest that the sulfur from the sulfate attachment may have some benefits of its own.[9] Because I recommend glucosamine be used with chondroitin sulfate, people taking both are getting sufficient quantities of sulfur in any event.

Unfortunately, most of the commercial products that claim to contain glucosamine sulfate aren't actually using the same compound that was used in research. Of greater importance, as we shall see in chapter 6, many of the products on the market today—perhaps over 80 percent—do not contain sufficient quantities of either glucosamine hydrochloride or glucosamine sulfate.

We do know for certain that N-acetyl glucosamine is not as effective in helping the cartilage cells produce more proteoglycans.[10] Because there's no clinical evidence that it works, products containing N-acetyl glucosamine should be avoided. Buyers should also be wary of products that claim to contain "glucosamine complex." Sometimes manufacturers mix the forms of glucosamine, perhaps thinking that this somehow sounds better to the consumer. What actually happens is that the dose of the different forms is far less than what has been shown to have an effect. Adding N-acetyl glucosamine may dilute the mixture so much that it doesn't work at all. For now, stick with glucosamine sulfate or glucosamine hydrochloride. New research may change this—you'll find updates on my Web site at www.drtheo.com.

The Proof Is in the Research

Theoretically, glucosamine should be a powerful osteoarthritis remedy. But theory and actual practice do not always agree, which is why theories are put to the test in controlled studies. Let's take a look at some of those studies—and see why glucosamine passed with flying colors.

As you read about these studies, bear in mind that the gold standard for medical research is a large, long-term, double-blind, placebo-controlled study. This type of study design reduces the possibility that the results are due to chance or bias. Since no one knows until the study is completed who is getting the placebo (an inactive substance such as a sugar pill) and who is receiving the real thing, the outcomes are not influenced by hope or bias by the researchers or participants.

The studies that show glucosamine/chondroitin works follow the gold standard. In fact, they go beyond it. To verify the results that individual studies show, researchers often use a technique called a meta-analysis. By applying powerful statistical tools to the combined results of a number of high-quality studies, a meta-analysis reveals the larger picture. In the case of glucosamine and chondroitin, meta-analysis has confirmed what we already knew: Glucosamine and chondroitin work.

If anyone tries to tell you that there isn't any scientific evidence for the effectiveness of glucosamine and chondroitin, be very skeptical. In fact, these supplements are among the most carefully researched therapies in all of osteoarthritis treatment. The kind and quality of the studies has equaled or exceeded that of the prescription and over-the-counter anti-inflammatory drugs you see advertised on TV and elsewhere. Not only has the research proved the benefit for relief of pain and improving function, but there is now substantial evidence showing that each of these supplements actually modifies and improves the disease process, something not possible with traditional pain relievers.

So many studies have been performed since the last edition of *The Arthritis Cure* that there isn't room to print them all here—I'll have to stick to some samples of ones that have appeared recently in prestigious medical journals. (If you would like to see the abstracts of these studies or print a copy for your physician to review, please visit my Web site at www.DrTheo.com.)

Let's start with one of the most important recent studies. In a randomized, double-blind, placebo-controlled trial, 212 patients with knee osteoarthritis were given 1,500 mg sulfate oral glucosamine or placebo once daily for three years. To determine the effect on the disease process, weight-bearing X rays of each knee were taken at the start and after one and three years to measure the width of the joint space (a sign of cartilage loss or gain). Symptoms of pain and function were assessed using a standard measure called the WOMAC score.

The 106 patients taking the placebo progressively lost joint space; after three years, the average joint space loss was 0.31 mm. There was no significant joint space loss in the 106 patients on glucosamine! Furthermore, pain and function worsened slightly in the patients taking the placebo, while a significant improvement was observed in the patients treated with glucosamine. There were no differences in the safety measures or reasons for withdrawing from the study when the placebo and glucosamine groups were compared. This fabulous study, published in the famed British medical journal *The Lancet* in 2001, shows that glucosamine, taken over the long term, was safe and effective at improving pain and function. Not only that, it modified the course of the disease, because the glucosamine group actually showed an improvement in pain and function.[11]

A very similar study done by different investigators with different patients confirmed the study discussed above. Here too, the study was a randomized, double-blind, placebo-controlled trial. Half of a group of 202 patients with knee osteoarthritis were given 1,500 mg oral glucosamine sulfate once daily for three years; the other group took a placebo once daily for three years. All the patients got regular X rays of their knees. The placebo group lost an average of 0.19 mm of joint space over the three-year period. The glucosamine group *gained* an average of 0.04 mm! In addition, the glucosamine group showed improvement in pain and function similar to that of full-dose, prescription anti-inflammatory medication—but without the potentially dangerous side effects of these drugs. Finally, the safety of long-term use was again confirmed. There was no significant difference in any of the standard safety measures, such as kidney function, liver function, cardiovascular problems, allergies, or any other measure evaluated.[12]

An early significant study looked at 80 patients in Milan, Italy, all suffering from severe, established osteoarthritis.[13] During the course of this 30-day double-blind study, the participants were given either 1.5 grams of glucosamine or a placebo.

Every week, the researchers took measurements of the patients' pain, joint tenderness, and swelling, as well as any restriction of active or passive movement. The final results were positive and exciting: The group treated with glucosamine experienced a significantly greater reduction in overall symptoms, compared to those who took the placebo (73 percent versus 41 percent).

It took only 20 days to reduce the symptoms by half in the glucosamine group, compared to 36 days for those who received the placebo.

A full 20 percent of the glucosamine-treated group became *completely symptom-free*, compared to *none* of the 40 patients on the placebo! When the physicians participating in the study were asked to rate the results, they reported that 29 out of the 40 glucosamine patients enjoyed "excellent" or "good" results, compared to only 17 of the 40 who received the placebo. Furthermore, when cartilage samples from the glucosamine-treated patients were examined under an electron microscope, they looked strikingly similar to healthy cartilage. But samples taken from the placebo group showed typical evidence of osteoarthritis. In other words, their cartilage looked "sick." The researchers concluded that glucosamine sulfate *rebuilt damaged cartilage*, thereby restoring function in most of the osteoarthritic patients taking the supplement.

Glucosamine has certainly shown its value in a number of studies. But how does it compare to popular pain remedies? So far, there have been four head-to-head comparisons in four controlled trials between glucosamine and prescription-strength anti-inflammatory drugs. In two of the studies, glucosamine equaled the ability of anti-inflammatories to reduce pain and improve function. The other two studies showed that glucosamine was better than the anti-inflammatories for relieving pain and improving function.[14] In all cases, glucosamine was deemed safer, as indicated by fewer adverse events or side effects. Furthermore, when patients were followed after discontinuation of glucosamine and the comparison drug, the people taking glucosamine were able to maintain their improvement in pain and function—but those taking the anti-inflammatories drifted back toward the pain and function problems they had at the beginning of the study. This is a testament to the fact that glucosamine is not only long-acting, but appears to improve the disease process itself, rather than just covering up the pain.

What you don't see in these studies, however, are the differences in the effects on the cartilage. None of these four studies actually looked at disease modification, so the true superiority of glucosamine over the anti-inflammatory drugs was not even highlighted. These were simply studies looking at pain and function in osteoarthritis sufferers. Here's an example of two of these studies.

Researchers in Portugal pitted glucosamine sulfate against ibuprofen (such as Advil®, Motrin®, and Nuprin®) in patients with osteoarthritis of the knee.[15] In this double-blind study, 40 patients were given a total of either 1.5 grams of glucosamine sulfate or 1.2 grams of ibuprofen daily (the same as taking six over-the-counter pills) over an eight-week period.

The pain levels dropped significantly in both groups during the first two weeks; in fact, the ibuprofen group enjoyed even quicker pain relief than the glucosamine group did. But after the first two weeks, the ibuprofen seemed to lose some of its strength and the pain relief began to fade. Glucosamine, on the other hand, continued strong throughout the treatment period. At the end of the eight-week period there was a dramatic difference in the pain scores between the groups. On a scale of 0 to 3, with 3 being most painful, the glucosamine group had a pain score of only 0.8, compared to the ibuprofen group's 2.2. Additionally, swelling of the knee stopped in 20 percent of the patients in the glucosamine group, compared to none in the ibuprofen group. Overall, 29 percent more patients in the glucosamine group had a good outcome.

Glucosamine was also pitted against ibuprofen by scientists from four laboratories, three German and one Italian.[16] Once again, glucosamine proved to be as effective as ibuprofen in controlling pain—and was much better tolerated. Of the 100 patients in the ibuprofen group, 35 complained of adverse effects throughout the treatment, with seven dropping out of the study altogether. But only six of the 100 patients in the glucosamine group experienced adverse effects, and only one dropped out.

Many glucosamine studies are done with patients who have knee arthritis, in large part because this joint is affected so often that there is a large pool of people to draw on. It's also fairly easy to X-ray the knee to see the changes in the joint space. That doesn't mean glucosamine is helpful only for knee arthritis, however—any joint with arthritis can be helped. In a 2001 study that appeared in the *Journal of the American Medical Association*, for instance, glucosamine was shown to be superior to ibuprofen for patients with arthritis in the temporomandibular joint (the "hinge" of the jaw). The conclusion after a three-month study of 45 patients? Glucosamine had a significantly greater influence in reducing pain produced during function (such as chewing) and effect of pain with daily activities. In addition, the study showed that glucosamine has a carryover effect. The study lasted for 90 days; after 120 days, the glucosamine patients needed far less pain medication than the ibuprofen group.[17]

Studies Show What Patients Know

It's not just those lucky enough to participate in university studies who enjoy the benefits of glucosamine. Many individuals are delighted at the relief they get upon taking the supplement. Sixty-two-year-old Edna Taylor enjoyed being active. After working as a part-time church volunteer every weekday morning, this cheerful woman tended her large garden and strolled in the afternoon. While getting into her car one evening, she noticed a small "twinge" in her right hip. "It was nothing," she explained later. "Just like someone gently pinched me."

A week later, the "gentle pinch" felt more like a vise clamping down on her right hip and upper leg. "When I walked, or even moved my leg, it felt like someone was hitting me there with a hammer! I couldn't do anything," she said. "No gardening, no walking. Just getting out of the chair to go to the bathroom was torture. I was really angry. Why did I get this? And why couldn't the doctors do anything?"

Not only did she have the original pain, she also soon suffered from headaches, blurred vision, and liver damage, all side effects of the various drugs her doctors prescribed. "Life used to be fun," she said dejectedly. "Now it's hell."

Fortunately, the situation improved when Edna began taking glucosamine. "I didn't notice anything for the first week. I thought it wasn't going to work and I decided to stop taking it at the end of Day 9. But when I woke up on Day 10, my hip felt a little better. So I kept taking it. On Day 15 it was 25 percent better, and on Day 20 it was 50 percent better. I called my sister to tell her it was 50 percent better, and she didn't believe me."

After taking the supplement for several weeks she was able to tend to her garden and stroll around the neighborhood as much as she had before. And she no longer had to worry about the powerful side effects of standard pain medications.

Don Summers, a 43-year-old world-class bicyclist, came to my office because he was still experiencing constant pain and swelling in his knee when bicycling, despite reconstructive ligament surgery. His knee just never seemed right after that. Anti-inflammatory medicines and applications of ice weren't working and, unable to exercise and train, Don became very depressed. But within a few weeks of taking glucosamine/chondroitin, Don really noticed a difference. Years later, he is 100 percent cured—there is absolutely no pain or swelling. In fact, he showed off his newfound health by giving me a piggyback ride as he jogged down two flights of stairs!

Glucosamine, standing alone, is a fabulous tool for relieving arthritis symptoms and restoring cartilage health. But the relief it brings is further enhanced by the use of a second nutritional supplement—chondroitin sulfate.

Chondroitin: The "Water Magnet"

Perhaps because people abbreviate glucosamine/chondroitin as "glucosamine," chondroitin often gets second billing. This is unfortunate, because the evidence for chondroitin exceeded that for glucosamine for many years. Only recently has the publication of new glucosamine studies evened out the tally. Chondroitin has many beneficial functions for joint health. Some overlap with glucosamine; some are unique. That's why I almost always recommend using them in tandem for a one-two punch against osteoarthritis.

Both glucosamine and chondroitin help to form the proteoglycans that sit within the spaces in the cartilage "netting." But chondroitin, a long chain of repeating sugars, acts like a "liquid magnet" and helps attract fluid into the proteoglycan molecules. This is important for two reasons: First, the fluid acts as a spongy shock absorber. Second, the fluid sweeps nutrients into the cartilage. Articular (joint) cartilage has no blood supply, so all of its nourishment and lubrication comes from the liquid that ebbs and flows as pressure to the joint is applied and released. Without this fluid, cartilage would become malnourished, drier, thinner, and more fragile.[18] When that happens, as a result, the cartilage cells eventually die off, leading to a slow but steady downhill degeneration of the cartilage and the joint as a whole.

How does chondroitin ensure that the proteoglycans will attract and hold water in the cartilage? It has to do with the structure of the chondroitin "chains." Imagine the tall, strong trunk of a tree stretching into the sky. This is the backbone of a proteoglycan molecule. Jutting out from this trunk are large branches (core proteins), and growing from each branch are 100 smaller branches (chondroitin sulfate chains). These chondroitin chains have negative electrical charges, which means they repel each other. Think of placing two magnets next to each other. If you align them with the opposite poles facing each other, the magnets attract. But if you align them with the same poles facing each other, they repel: The magnets don't want to be pushed together. The negative charges of chondroitin work the same way, pushing chondroitins apart, thus creating a space that forms the matrix of the cartilage. There may be as many as 10,000 of these chains in just a single proteoglycan molecule, making it a super water retainer!

You're probably already getting very small amounts of chondroitin from your diet. It's found in most animal tissues, especially in the gristle around joints. I have often theorized that our intake of chondroitin was much greater in the past. I'm sure our Stone Age ancestors ate all the ligaments, tendons, and capsules around the joints of animals they killed, and probably also ate the cartilage on the ends of the bones. Today, few of us eat these parts, so the dietary intake of chondroitin has probably declined over the years. Fortunately, supplementing with oral chondroitin is proven to work. Some of the chondroitins we eat are absorbed into our bodies intact and incorporated into various tissues, including articular cartilage. In fact, carefully controlled absorption studies have shown that about 12 to 15 percent of the chondroitin you take by mouth is actually absorbed into the body.[19]

This compares to about 85 percent absorption for glucosamine. Don't let these numbers fool you in to thinking glucosamine's effect is better just because it's better absorbed. Chondroitin has a special affinity or attraction to osteoarthritic cartilage, so it tends to concentrate in the cartilage that needs the most help.[20] This sets it apart from glucosamine and balances out the differences in absorption. You could even argue that the *effective* absorption of chondroitin, as a result of the special affinity, is *higher* than glucosamine. Because of that, we can use a somewhat smaller dose of chondroitin (800 to 1,200 mg) compared to glucosamine (1,500 mg).

ABSORPTION RATES AND REALITY

Don't let the supplement marketers fool you with the term "absorption." The amount absorbed for any supplement or drug has very little to do with its effectiveness. One of the most powerful drugs for improving bone density, alendronate (Fosamax®), has an absorption of only about 0.6 percent. In other words, over 99 percent of it never gets into the body. The absorption rate for chondroitin is about 25 times greater than this. Absorption just tells us the dosage we should consider, not the effectiveness of the product.

The Role of Chondroitin

Besides drawing in precious fluid, chondroitin has other crucial functions in your joints:

- It protects existing cartilage from premature breakdown by inhibiting the action of certain cartilage-chewing enzymes.[21]
- It helps prevent the age-related death of chondrocytes.[22]
- It stimulates the production of proteoglycans, glycosaminoglycans, and collagen, the cartilage matrix molecules that serve as building blocks for healthy new cartilage.[23]
- Chondroitin increases the synthesis of hyaluronan, which can make the joint fluid thicker and help it be a better shock absorber.[24]
- Chondroitin inhibits the negative effects of interleukin-1 beta (IL-1b) and blocks Tumor Necrosis Factor alpha (TNF-alpha).[25] IL-1b and TNF-alpha are involved in cartilage destruction.
- Chondroitin shows a mild anti-inflammatory effect[26] and can reduce the need for anti-inflammatory drugs.[27]
- It works synergistically with glucosamine—each substance enhances the action of the other.[28]

Fortunately, supplemental chondroitin works very much like the naturally occurring chondroitin in your cartilage, protecting the old cartilage from premature breakdown and stimulating the synthesis of new cartilage.

A review article published in 2000 on nine double-blind and placebo-controlled chondroitin studies showed how safe this supplement is. The studies indicated no serious adverse effects from chondroitin, and there were fewer minor side effects than even in the placebo groups![29] This means that we don't have to suffer when our natural healthy cartilage mechanisms break down. We can replace with supplements what our bodies fail to make or don't make in sufficient amounts.

Chondroitin Research

Just like glucosamine, chondroitin has been put to the test in hospitals and research centers. The results have been surprisingly positive and encouraging.

In 2001, Swiss, French, and American researchers teamed up to evaluate 300 patients with documented osteoarthritis of the knee. A double-blind, randomized, placebo-controlled study utilized 800 mg of chondroitin in the treatment group. This was a long-term study (two years in duration) designed to prove that chondroitin had disease-modifying effects on osteoarthritis. Careful X-ray analysis before and after the intervention revealed that subjects in the placebo group lost cartilage at the expected rate, but the group treated with chondroitin had no significant change over the two years. This difference was statistically significant and offered very convincing evidence for the 800 mg daily dose of chondroitin.[30]

Another, even larger two-year X-ray study presented in 2003 using 800 mg of chondroitin per day showed that the minimal joint space width increased in the knees of the chondroitin users while dropping significantly in the placebo group. More impressive, this happened independent of whether or not there was any pain reduction noticed by the study subjects![31]

How did these results compare to using prescription anti-inflammatory drugs? In chapter 7, we will describe a study using rofe-coxib (Vioxx®) that showed dramatic losses in the cartilage over only one year of treatment. Pain and function studies also significantly favor chondroitin, not only for safety and side effects, but because chondroitin users have greater improvements in pain and function for a prolonged period of time, even after the chondroitin is no longer taken.

A double-blind, randomized study performed in France in 1992 compared the painkilling effectiveness of chondroitin sulfate to a placebo.[32] For this study, 120 patients with osteoarthritis of the knees and hips were given either oral chondroitin or a placebo. In addition, all the patients received the same doses of NSAIDs. At the end of three months, the patients taking chondroitin showed a significant improvement in pain and function. The chondroitin was very well tolerated by all who took it—no patients had to withdraw prematurely from the study due to side effects. As an added bonus, there was a carryover effect: the patients in the chondroitin group continued to experience the benefits during the two-month post-treatment evaluation phase of the study. Every study on chondroitin that looked for a post-treatment effect has shown that the benefits of pain reduction and improved function continued, even months after stopping the chondroitin. One study showed that the benefit of pain reduction continued to improve to lower and lower levels, even though the chondroitin was stopped two months earlier. Chondroitin appears to have a much longer residual affect than glucosamine or any other oral treatment for osteoarthritis. In fact, when researchers do studies in osteoarthritis now, they try to make sure that the study subjects haven't been using glucosamine for at least the previous two to three months, or chondroitin for the previous four to six months (this is called a washout period). They have to do this to prevent influencing the study results by having residual effects from the glucosamine or chondroitin—and because the supplements are so popular, they often have trouble finding volunteers who aren't already using them or are willing to give them up.

The effects of chondroitin might actually be much longer than six months. The researchers picked this timeframe somewhat arbitrarily, because nobody has really followed people after they've discontinued chondroitin for more than two months. By contrast, the washout period for users of acetaminophen and anti-inflammatory drugs is usually only a few days, a testament to the fact that these drugs are only pain relievers and don't do much, if anything, to improve joint health.

Real-world proof shows that chondroitin is not only an effective treatment for osteoarthritis, it's also a *cost-effective* treatment. A study in France looked at how well chondroitin reduced patients' reliance on anti-inflammatory drugs to treat the pain of osteoarthritis. The study looked at some 11,000 patients; some were being seen by primary care physicians, some by arthritis specialists. Those patients taking 1,200 mg of chondroitin daily used 63 percent *less* anti-inflammatory medication overall. For the subgroup seeing specialists, the results were even more remarkable: 85 percent less anti-inflammatory medication was required. Of course, these numbers are averages. Some patients were able to decrease their anti-inflammatory intake only slightly, but some were able to completely eliminate the need for the drugs, in itself a huge victory in treating osteoarthritis![33] Because anti-inflammatory medications can cost *three times* or more than a daily dose of chondroitin, this data alone showed that chondroitin is cost-effective. But when you consider that the use of anti-inflammatory medications often requires the use of other medicines to help offset adverse side effects, along with the fact that over one hundred thousand Americans a year are hospitalized from the complications of these drugs, it's easy to see that chondroitin more than pays for itself.

The magnitude of the cost-reduction was determined in another European study. One hundred osteoarthritis patients who were all using anti-inflammatory drugs to control pain were assigned to randomly receive either chondroitin or a prescription anti-inflammatory drug. The patients were evaluated for pain and function and were followed for one year. Even though the anti-inflammatory drug was available as a generic and was inexpensive, the overall cost to treat the patients with osteoarthritis was 49.1 percent *lower* in those receiving the chondroitin. Furthermore, the chondroitin users enjoyed better control of their pain and had improved function compared to those receiving the anti-inflammatory drugs.[34] It's no wonder that some European countries will partially or fully subsidize patients who are prescribed chondroitin for treatment of their osteoarthritis. The overall costs are lower, the pain and function improvement is better, and the safety is unsurpassed for those using the chondroitin. Consider this if you balk at paying a relatively high price for quality supplements!

As of 2003, there had been about 40 controlled clinical human studies on glucosamine and chondroitin. At least sixteen of these studies have been double-blind and placebo-controlled. I don't have space here to look at all sixteen, but two different summary reviews of these studies have been published. In one of the reviews, the overall treatment effect of chondroitin actually exceeded that for glucosamine; in the other, both were considered to have similar positive effects on the improvement in pain and function of osteoarthritis patients.[35]

The good news gets even better. These studies and reviews looked at glucosamine and chondroitin separately. When taken together, the effects are even more encouraging.

Glucosamine/Chondroitin: The One-Two Punch

Something apparently goes wrong with the cartilage matrix in a person with osteoarthritis. The body doesn't produce proteoglycans and collagen, the building blocks of cartilage, fast enough to keep the cartilage healthy. (This is one of the effects that aging has on cartilage.) At the same time, cartilage-chewing enzymes are hard at work, destroying the working cartilage that is present. It's a two-part problem that needs a two-part solution: glucosamine *and* chondroitin. Used together, glucosamine and chondroitin enhance cartilage repair and improve joint function.

Working together synergistically, glucosamine/chondroitin stimulate the synthesis of new cartilage while simultaneously keeping the cartilage-busting enzymes under control and the chondrocytes healthy. This helps to normalize the cartilage matrix, in essence treating the disease at the cellular level. Other arthritis treatments relieve pain or reduce inflammation, but don't touch the underlying problem in the cartilage. The one-two punch of glucosamine/chondroitin can actually halt the disease process in its tracks and help the body heal itself.

By itself, each supplement is effective. Together, they may well be the answer for millions of people suffering from osteoarthritis, the solution that works where drugs and surgeries have failed. A number of scientific articles have been written to explain why these substances work better when taken together. To put it briefly, in order to qualify as a truly chondroprotective agent, a compound must be able to:

1. enhance cartilage cell macromolecule synthesis (glycosaminoglycans, proteoglycans, collagens, proteins, RNA, and DNA)
2. enhance the synthesis of hyaluronan (the substance that gives the joint fluid its thick viscosity, providing lubrication between the synovial membrane and cartilage)

3. inhibit the enzymes that degrade the cartilage cell macromolecules
4. remove blood clots, fat deposits, and cholesterol deposits from within the synovial spaces and blood vessels in surrounding joints
5. reduce joint pain
6. reduce synovitis (swelling of the synovial membrane)
7. help prevent the early death of cartilage cells (chondrocytes)

No drug or supplement acting alone can do all that. But glucosamine and chondroitin working together can and do. Clinical and basic science studies have shown that glucosamine can accomplish objectives 1, 2, 3, 5, and 6, while chondroitin handles numbers 1, 2, 3, 4, 5, and 7. Their overlapping abilities explain why the glucosamine and chondroitin combination is such a powerful one-two punch against osteoarthritis.

A sophisticated study in 2000 proved the superiority of the combination by looking at cartilage samples before and after treatment with the supplements alone or together, compared to a placebo. The results confirmed the theory first proposed in the original edition of *The Arthritis Cure*. Glucosamine and chondroitin alone were significantly more effective than the placebo group in preventing erosions of the cartilage. But the combination of glucosamine and chondroitin was able to prevent the most severe cartilage erosions, and was able to synergistically increase the production of proteoglycans from cartilage cells.[36]

The NIH GAIT Study

My main reason for developing the Arthritis Cure treatment program was to give the public a solution to the number-one cause of chronic pain and disability. In addition, I wanted to save lives by allowing people a substitute for dangerous anti-inflammatory medications and surgery. It was then, and it is today, very difficult to know that thousands of people are needlessly dying or suffering from the adverse consequences of the traditional treatments for osteoarthritis when we have something so much better and safer. The Arthritis Cure was the first complete program that actually was disease-modifying for osteoarthritis. From an academic perspective, however, I had the additional goal of raising awareness about these fantastic supplements in an effort to stimulate more research.

It was a great honor and pleasure in 2002 to be asked to be on the Steering Oversight Committee for the $16 million National Institutes of Health (NIH) study of glucosamine and chondroitin. The official name of the study is GAIT, for Glucosamine/Chondroitin Arthritis Intervention Trial.

The aim of this study is to add to the already impressive body of research related to the supplements by analyzing information on the largest single group of subjects to date.

The study is designed to be simultaneously performed at several research institutions. It is double-blinded and placebo-controlled and looks at several factors related to the supplements, including safety and tolerability.

Over 1,500 study subjects will be split into five groups, or arms:

Arm 1: Orally administered glucosamine HCL alone (1,500 mg)
Arm 2: Orally administered chondroitin sulfate alone (1,200 mg)
Arm 3: Combination of glucosamine and chondroitin
Arm 4: The anti-inflammatory drug celecoxib (Celebrex®)
Arm 5: Placebo

The study really has two different parts. The major part of the study looks at pain and function parameters over a six-month period of treatment. A smaller subset of subjects will be evaluated for potential disease-modifying effects (ability to prevent loss of cartilage) in the five treatment arms over a two-year period. Disease-modifying effects will be evaluated by weight-bearing knee X rays taken before and after the two-year intervention.

The estimated completion date for the study is about 2005. The investigators have had a hard time recruiting study subjects. It is difficult to find arthritis patients who meet all of the rigorous criteria to participate in the study, including those who are not already taking glucosamine and chondroitin, and those who are willing to be randomly put into a placebo group (or a group that is just taking Celebrex®).

Despite the tremendous effort by all the researchers involved in the study, this trial, like all trials, is not perfect. Most of the imperfections are due not to any of the researchers' efforts, but to the technical limitations of measuring cartilage loss. Unfortunately, I expect some of these imperfections to either diminish the true benefit of the supplements or, in the worst case, even change the entire conclusion of the study.

The most significant problems with the study are related to the portion that looks at changes in the cartilage width before and after treatment with each of the five arms. As mentioned earlier, X rays are not very sensitive in detecting the very small loss of cartilage that occurs in people with osteoarthritis. In fact, the loss of cartilage in several studies has averaged approximately 0.1 mm per year in the knees, though some studies show a higher loss.

GAIT will be assessing study subjects by X ray over a two-year period. If the averages hold, we would expect those people taking the placebo to lose about 0.2 mm of cartilage in their knees.

Even if people in the glucosamine and chondroitin groups are able to *increase* the cartilage in their joints by 0.1 mm, however, the way this study is designed, this might not be considered a *significant* difference from a statistical standpoint. Because of the crudeness of the X-ray techniques, nothing less than perhaps a 0.2 mm difference may be considered significant.

Even without having any knowledge whatsoever about the results of the study (no one does yet, since we are all blinded to the results until the end), it would be a good bet to predict that *no* treatment arm will be able to show such a dramatic change in the cartilage in such a short time.

Because the bar is being placed so high, the almost inevitable overall conclusion will be that glucosamine and chondroitin had no effect as disease-modifying agents. The headlines in the media will no doubt say "Glucosamine and chondroitin have no effect on cartilage," even if this is not quite the truth. After all, we know from three other large, long-term studies and three smaller studies that people taking the supplements do show a significant benefit as determined by X ray. Animal studies, where we can actually look at the cartilage under the microscope before and after treatment and detect changes and improvements in the cartilage, show the same thing. And because animal studies look inside the joint, they are far more accurate than the relatively crude method of using X rays.

The potentially tragic conclusion to the GAIT study could damage the credibility of these supplements, even though they have been shown in several other disease-modifying studies (of a duration up to *three* years) to significantly modify the osteoarthritis disease process by halting loss of cartilage.

As one veteran osteoarthritis researcher told me, "I don't even know why they're doing this part of the study; we know what the results are going to be." We went on to compare this to trying to determine who could jump higher, a lion or a pig. Suppose both animals are placed behind a 20-foot brick wall and you waited on the other side to observe them as they came over the top. When neither appears on the other side because neither can jump 20 feet, you still can't assume that the animals have equal jumping ability. The wall was too high for either animal to clear.

This is the same problem we face with determining the disease-modifying effect in the NIH study. The pigs (celecoxib and placebo) could get the same billing as the lions (glucosamine and chondroitin).

The disease-modifying portion of the study can be repaired, however, by either adding larger numbers of people and then following them for a longer period of time, or by using a more sensitive detection device or method. This would cost more money to do, but there's a lot at stake. Americans are spending over $80 billion a year in direct and indirect costs from osteoarthritis and the results of this trial will be viewed as critical.

If the study population in the placebo group loses cartilage at a much faster rate than 0.1 mm per year, a significant difference in disease modification may become apparent, even if the investigators don't change any features of the study. The investigators are committed to making GAIT as accurate and cost-effective as possible.

As updates on the study and the final results become available, I'll post the information on my Web site at www.drtheo.com.

If Glucosamine/Chondroitin Are So Good . . .

The theory is sound and the studies are good. So why aren't more doctors using glucosamine/chondroitin? The reason is a complicated mix of medical conservatism, consumer attitudes, and commercial reality. Throughout their four years of medical school, plus several years more of residency and possibly further training, many physicians are taught that drugs and surgery are the "best" ways to treat patients. Some medical students take a course in nutrition, but the bulk of them receive little or no nutritional/dietary training at all. That's why so many doctors scoff at the mere mention of glucosamine/chondroitin—they're not interested because they don't know any better.

The big pharmaceutical companies weren't interested in glucosamine or chondroitin sulfate either, at least not until millions of people started using them. Drug companies like to put their money into products they can patent, like drugs. The patent protects their product, allowing them to corner the market and make a lot of money. Since they can't patent most supplements, they don't want to work with them. They don't invest money to study the supplements, and they don't flood doctors' offices with free samples or information as they do with their drugs. In fact, a new trend has occurred in the pharmaceutical industry. Part of the multibillion-dollar research and development budget that some companies enjoy is devoted to performing studies on competitive products in an effort to try to discredit them, indirectly helping their own product in the process. Some of the research articles that they publish have been criticized as having significant bias, some companies have tried to withhold negative information that has been uncovered, and some have been publicly chastised for purposefully manipulating the interpretation of study data (including that for Celebrex®, a pain reliever). There have been well-documented cases of this occurring not only against competitive pharmaceutical products in the same category, but also supplements that may interfere with the sales of patented drugs.

Because annual sales of dietary supplements top $18 billion in the

United States, however, the pharmaceutical companies have started to take notice of the dietary supplement industry. At least two pharmaceutical companies have ventured into the glucosamine/chondroitin arena. The maker of Tylenol® sells a product that not only contains an unproven mixture of glucosamine but is about 30 percent below the well-established effective daily glucosamine dosage. Despite its lack of full potency, this is one of the most expensive glucosamine products on the market. Another company sells a mixture of glucosamine and chondroitin that, to the amazement of many, failed an independent analysis of its label claim—the pills did not contain the amounts listed on the label.

As with most dramatic medical advances, it takes time for revolutionary information to make its way into the minds of health professionals and eventually to the public. Fortunately, this process is now well under way, for several reasons:

- Thanks to new research on the genesis of osteoarthritis, more and more doctors are realizing that osteoarthritis is not an inevitable part of growing older. Normal wear and tear is not the problem. Instead, problems with the cartilage matrix are to blame—breakdown is exceeding build-up. Armed with this new understanding, physicians are beginning to look for a way to "fix" the matrix. They are finally realizing that cartilage loss is not a one-way, downhill event.
- With the increasing internationalization of the drug and health-food industries, American doctors are learning more about European research into cartilage repair and regeneration.
- Doctors have a greater general awareness of the healing powers of many nutritional supplements. As more high-quality research is performed, doctors can't help but embrace the findings.
- More and more physicians, including many leaders in the area of arthritis treatment, are becoming aware of the value of glucosamine/chondroitin. They've been hearing about it from their patients, and even seeing for themselves how well it works. Positive studies showing that these supplements work have appeared in widely read, highly prestigious medical journals, and

well-informed, thought-leading doctors have spoken out in favor of them.

Physicians are getting the message. A small but growing number are starting to recommend supplements as part of their treatment protocols, without awaiting for official acknowledgment from the medical establishment.

The change is beginning. I believe that in the near future physicians across the country will be prescribing glucosamine/chondroitin for most or all of their osteoarthritis patients on a regular basis.

Where Can I Get Glucosamine and Chondroitin?

Glucosamine/chondroitin can be purchased without a prescription from a variety of sources, including health-food stores, pharmacies, and even grocery stores. The supplements are marketed under different brand names, with different strengths and levels of purity, and not all of them are high-quality products. This is in an area that may be just as important to understand as the use and research related to the supplements.

Before rushing out to buy glucosamine/chondroitin, please study chapter 6 carefully. You'll learn how to select high-quality products, how much of each supplement to take, special considerations, and how to use the supplements as the spearhead of the nine-step Arthritis Cure. And remember: You don't need a prescription for glucosamine or chondroitin, but as always, you should speak with your physician before beginning to use these supplements.

As you get ready to implement the Arthritis Cure using glucosamine and chondroitin, be sure to also read the next chapter to learn about ASU, an exciting new addition to the arsenal of arthritis-fighting supplements.

─4─
ASU: ADDING TO THE ARSENAL

What is ASU?

How does ASU work?

Is there good evidence for this supplement?

Where can I get ASU?

The dawn of a new era in the treatment of osteoarthritis has arrived. In January 1997 I introduced you to glucosamine and chondroitin and my revolutionary nine-step treatment program for osteoarthritis. Glucosamine and chondroitin were the first disease-modifying intervention for arthritis, and introducing them forever changed the way we treat the number-one cause of chronic pain in America.

A year later, I introduced you to SAMe, a natural treatment for depression and an additional treatment for the pain of osteoarthritis. SAMe has now been proven in a government report to be safe and effective.[1] (For more about SAMe and arthritis, please check chapter 10.)

Since then, these supplements and the nine-step treatment program have proven themselves again and again, helping millions of people worldwide. Large, well-conducted research studies from around the world and review articles in major medical journals have verified that the treatment works better and is safer than the drug treatments prescribed most often.

I am very proud to help arthritis treatment make another important leap forward by introducing a new, proven, innovative therapy that will help broaden the scope of the Arthritis Cure. Glucosamine and chondroitin have helped millions; I believe the new treatment will help millions more.

ASU: Avocado Soybean Unsaponifiables

A natural vegetable extract made from avocado and soybean oils, avocado soybean unsaponifiables has been a prescription treatment for osteoarthritis in France since the early 1990s. In the research literature, the cumbersome term *avocado soybean unsaponifiables* is abbreviated as ASU.

ASU has been so well studied, and so well accepted, that the French national health insurance program (widely considered the finest in the world) has, for many years, partially or fully reimbursed French citizens who were prescribed it for the treatment of their osteoarthritis. France has long been ahead of the United States in osteoarthritis treatment—prescription chondroitin was used there for many years prior to its introduction into the U.S. In fact, several of the chondroitin studies and almost all of the ASU studies originated with French researchers and universities.

ASU differs from glucosamine and chondroitin, and all other treatments for osteoarthritis, in that it is a mixture of many different plant substances—it is not just one compound or molecule. ASU is not the same thing as avocado oil, an expensive, flavorful oil used mostly for salad dressings; it's also not the same as inexpensive soybean oil used as a cooking oil. Rather, ASU comes from a very small fraction of the natural oil found in avocados and soybeans; the supplement is mixed in a ratio of one part avocado to two parts soybean. The processing to get ASU from its sources is very complex. Raw, fresh avocados and soybeans are cleaned and mashed and then undergo a series of processing steps to extract the desired portions of the oil without damaging the active components—which is by no means easy to do. This oil is then highly refined in a lengthy series of additional steps to get the finished product. Careful controls are required at every one of the production stages. The exact details of the processing are patented or proprietary, but even from this brief description it's easy to see that the procedure to make ASU is costly and time-consuming.

Not only is sophisticated processing required, but material selection is critical as well. For instance, if avocados are not used at the right stage of maturity, the concentration of key ingredients can vary several-fold.[2]

A large quantity of raw material—fresh avocados and soybeans—is needed to make ASU. Only a fraction of whole avocados and soybeans is made up of oil and of that oil, only a tiny fraction is the unsaponifiable portion. There's so little ASU in a single avocado or handful of soybeans that you couldn't possibly eat enough of them to get a useful dose of ASU; only the supplements contain enough to be therapeutically useful. There's another limiting factor: Not only is ASU a very tiny component of raw avocados and soybeans, it's bound up by plant fibers that inhibit absorption in the human digestive system. Even if you ate really large quantities of avocados and soybeans, you'd not be able to absorb enough ASU to have a significant benefit on the health of your joints.

It's pretty clear where the words avocado and soybean come from in ASU, but what exactly does *unsaponifiable* mean? *Saponify* is a chemical term that literally means "to make soap." *Unsaponifiable* means that this fraction of the avocado/soybean oil cannot be congealed into a solid in the same way that other types of fats and oils are processed into soap by the addition of lye. Unsaponifiable is a general descriptive term used in chemistry to categorize this component of plant oils.

Since ASU is a mixture of many different types of plant compounds, no one to date has been able to identify exactly which components are most important. Based on the research that has been done with individual components, however, the bulk of the evidence points toward *phytosterols,* a natural group of fatty substances found in all plants, as the active ingredients in ASU. In fact, ASU is also sometimes called ASP, for avocado soy phytosterols. Also present in ASU are the *tocopherols,* the family of compounds that include the many forms of vitamin E, although these substances probably play only a minor role. Some other very complex, specific components in the avocado are probably of significance as well. Research in this area is very active, and more definitive answers about ASU's active ingredients should be available within the next few years.

The Importance of Phytosterols

Also known as plant sterols or sterolins, phytosterols are fats found in all plants, including fruits and vegetables. Phytosterols are to plant cells as cholesterol is to animal or human cells. The chemical structure is similar but the effects are quite different. In fact, eating a lot of phytosterols can lower cholesterol levels. As I'll discuss below, supplementing your diet with phytosterols can provide significant health benefits for a whole host of conditions.

Just as we all have cholesterol in our blood, we all have phytosterols as well. The concentration of cholesterol outnumbers that of phytosterols by hundreds of times. Both are essential to good health. Even though we often equate cholesterol as being "bad," we couldn't survive without it. Cholesterol is a key component in the walls of all of our cells and is also used as the building block for certain hormones, including estrogen and testosterone. You don't need to *eat* cholesterol, however, because your liver will make it from various foods you eat. We do need to eat phytosterols, however—our bodies have no way to manufacture these substances from other foods. That's a major reason why nuts, fruits, vegetables, and plant oils are vital for good health. Epidemiologic evidence suggests that a higher intake of phytosterols is quite desirable. For instance, according to an article in the *Journal of the National Cancer Institute*, the typical Western diet contains 80 mg of phytosterols per day, whereas vegetarian and Japanese diets contain four to five times as much—345 mg per day and 400 mg per day, respectively.[3] Phytosterols are generally tightly bound to the various types of fiber found in plants. Since humans cannot digest most plant fibers, many of the phytosterols we eat pass through the digestive system without being absorbed.

Research on Phytosterols

Research on ASU dates back to the mid-1970s when it was used (and still is) as a treatment for periodontal (gum) disease in dentistry. It's also used to treat scleroderma, a connective tissue disorder treated by rheumatologists (see chapter 12 for more on this disease).[4]

The bulk of the current research on ASU, however, has been for the treatment of osteoarthritis. Phytosterols, which make up some of the main active components in ASU, are some of the better-researched plant substances. Interest in their beneficial effects on the human body has led to an explosion of research in just the past few years. Scientists have been able to quantify the concentration of phytosterols in various plant substances. Plant oils have the highest concentration; seeds and nuts are intermediate; lower levels are found in fruits and vegetables. By definition, animal products, including fish, are devoid of significant phytosterols.

The phytosterol family includes a number of different components. The most common phytosterols in the diet are beta-sitosterol, campesterol, and stigmasterol. These compounds are also key ingredients in processed ASU.

Much of the initial research interest on phytosterols was related to the prevention of heart disease. Increasing dietary intake, or providing supplementation, has been shown to have a significant benefit in lowering cholesterol.[5] Phytosterols accomplish this by blocking cholesterol absorption in the small intestine, causing dietary cholesterol to pass out of the body. (It's this effect that makes cholesterol-reducing spreads such as Benecol® work.)

In addition to the benefits to the cardiovascular system from ASU, a large amount of research looks at ASU for other areas as well, including cancer prevention and treatment,[6] immune system enhancement,[7] and for use in alleviating the symptoms of an enlarged prostate.[8]

Phytosterols can be isolated from a variety of plant oils and plant products. For the treatment of osteoarthritis, however, the key source is from the mixture of the unsaponifiable portion of avocado and soybean oils in a 1:2 ratio (one part avocado unsaponifiable to two parts soybean unsaponifiable oil). Lab research using human cartilage cells has also shown that the mixture of the two unsaponifiable fractions is more effective for treating arthritis than either fraction by itself.[9] Don't let people try to fool you into thinking that just any phytosterols will do the job in treating your osteoarthritis. And remember, other components in ASU likely confer activity for joint health as well—research in this area continues.

ASU and Osteoarthritis

The research evidence for ASU spans the full spectrum required to prove that it is an effective treatment for osteoarthritis. There is plentiful basic science research showing that ASU can act on both phases in the osteoarthritis process, increasing the stimulation of cartilage and decreasing its breakdown.

The same study that tells us both the avocado and soybean fractions are needed for the best results also gives us an important clue as to how ASU works: It seems to inhibit the production of some interleukins and other substances that are associated with increased inflammation. (Interleukins are natural chemicals your body produces as part of the immune response.) This helps prevent the breakdown of cartilage. Research has shown that both the production of specialized joint collagen and proteoglycans in the articular cartilage can be increased significantly by adding ASU to cartilage cultures.[10] In 2003, additional lab research showed that ASU stimulates the production of aggrecans (another name for proteoglycans) and reduces the production of interleukins and other pro-inflammatory substances.[11]

Taking the research to the next step, how it performs in a living system indicates that the basic science research in the lab is indeed valid. Research on animals shows that ASU can act as a chondroprotective agent, preventing the loss of cartilage when it is subjected to the sort of mechanical or chemical damage that is known to lead to osteoarthritis.

Human studies further validate ASU as a viable and safe treatment for osteoarthritis. The studies looked at the traditional indicators of success in a treatment for osteoarthritis, such as pain and function, and saw real improvement. The studies were so well performed, and so superior, that a review of all herbal therapies for osteoarthritis completed up to 2002 indicated that ASU was the only plant-based, oral treatment that had sufficient evidence to be recommended for general use in osteoarthritis.[12]

Finally, emerging data shows that ASU, like glucosamine and chondroitin, has disease-modifying properties in human osteoarthritis. This was shown by an important study in 2002. The study looked at 163 people with documented and painful osteoarthritis of the hip. The patients were entered into a prospective, randomized, double-blind, placebo-controlled study of two years' duration utilizing 300 mg of ASU or placebo. Neither the patients nor the researchers knew who was getting the real ASU and who was getting the dummy pills.

In the patients who had less severe osteoarthritis, there was no difference between ASU and placebo in preventing cartilage loss. But, to the surprise of the researchers, there was a significant difference when looking at those patients who had worse than average osteoarthritis of the hip. The placebo group had double the loss of hip joint space width (0.86 mm) compared to those using ASU (0.43 mm), showing that the arthritis of the people taking the placebo progressed more than the arthritis of the people taking the ASU. There were no significant differences in adverse effects between the ASU and placebo groups.

This study was important for several reasons. First of all, it confirmed that ASU is safe over a period of at least two years—although we already knew this because the supplement has been used for years in France. Second, it was effective in modifying the disease process among those who were severely affected. By comparison, most arthritis treatments work best in mild or moderate disease and don't help as much in severe disease. Because ASU has been shown to help in severe cases, it is a good candidate to use in conjunction with glucosamine and chondroitin for the treatment of osteoarthritis.[13]

One of the best aspects of ASU treatment is that it allows the majority of its users to significantly decrease their intake of NSAIDs if they'd been requiring these drugs for pain relief on a regular basis. Because of the dangers and toxicity of these drugs, anything that is safe and can reduce or eliminate a person's reliance on them should be considered a huge success. If we were able to get all Americans off NSAIDs, for instance, we could save over 16,500 lives per year. That's more than 45 people every day on average! Those figures are based on estimates done in 1998. I'm sure this figure would be even higher today, especially since the advertising and promotion of NSAIDs has increased exponentially over the past five years, and we now know that NSAIDs can block the beneficial effect of low-dose aspirin on the heart.

Let's look at an example of the research that showed ASU could reduce NSAIDs use. In this study, 260 people aged between 45 and 80 with documented osteoarthritis of the knees and taking regular NSAIDs were given either 300 mg or 600 mg of ASU or placebo in a double-blind, placebo-controlled trial lasting three months. Even though the duration of treatment was relatively short, there was a significant improvement in the measures of pain and function and a significant reduction in both the number of days taking NSAIDs as well as the overall dosages of NSAIDs required to control pain. In fact, NSAID and analgesic intake decrease by at least 50 percent in almost three quarters of those taking ASU—a statistically significant difference from placebo. The beneficial effects of the ASU were equal at the 300 mg and 600 mg dosages and began after the first month of therapy.

This excellent study provides further proof that 300 mg of ASU taken once a day for arthritis can relieve pain, improve function, and help break the dependence on NSAIDs.[14]

Finally, like glucosamine/chondroitin, the benefits of ASU continue even if you stop taking the supplements. This was shown by a major clinical trial of patients with painful hip or knee arthritis that went on for six months. Half the 164 patients received 300 mg of ASU daily; the other half got a dummy capsule. The ASU group showed significant improvement in pain and function; the placebo group didn't. At the end of the six months, both groups were given a placebo to see if the effect of ASU would continue even after the patients stopped taking it. It did—the positive effect continued for two more months.[15]

When ASU is added to glucosamine and chondroitin, which can also help break the reliance on NSAIDs, the effect should be even more powerful. ASU should become part of the first-line therapy for osteoarthritis, before NSAIDs or acetaminophen are even considered.

Side Effects, Safety Profile, and Use of ASU

Since ASU has been used as a pharmaceutical product in France for a number of years, the French government has required tracking of serious side effects or adverse reactions, much as the FDA does for prescription drugs in the United States. At this time, we are not aware of any known interactions with other medications or supplements, nor have any deaths been attributed to the use of ASU. Compare that to the anti-inflammatories, which interact badly with a wide range of drugs and are a major cause of emergency room visits by the elderly.

ASU is a vegetarian product. It is taken in a once-daily dose of 300 mg (active ingredients). It can be taken as a separate supplement or in combination with glucosamine and chondroitin. There have not been any studies to date combining all three supplements. We would expect, however, that adding ASU could provide additional symptom relief, and perhaps even add to the disease-modifying properties of glucosamine and chondroitin supplements.

ASU supplements are just beginning to be available on the American market, and it's too soon to say which products will be the best and which will need to be avoided—or even to provide the brand names of high-quality products. Right now, ASU supplements are on the expensive side, because the process to make the purified form is complex and difficult. Unfortunately, as with any other expensive supplement, there will doubtless be some unscrupulous companies that will try to sell you plain avocado or soybean oil and not the purified and highly refined, unsaponifiable fraction, or some unproven blend of phytosterols, under the guise of ASU. There may well also be manufacturers who will skimp on the amount of ASU in their products and not include at least 300 mg of active ingredient in each capsule.

To find the manufacturers who are making high-quality products, please check my Web site at www.drtheo.com. I'll be monitoring the ongoing research and providing the latest information and product evaluations as they become available. As I do for glucosamine and chondroitin, I'll also be tracking reports to me and to the FDA of adverse events and drug interactions.

—5—

THE ARTHRITIS CURE

The nine-step Arthritis Cure program.

*Current issues in the use of glucosamine,
chondroitin, and ASU.*

D ave Johnson, a 32-year-old salesman, was completely disgusted with the results of his two knee surgeries. "All I wanted was to be able to get around like a normal person, without that damn pain. But both surgeries were a real bust—they changed absolutely nothing. In my job in outside sales I'm in and out of the car maybe ten times a day, hauling my 25-pound case of samples in and out of office buildings. It's pretty demanding physically, even on a good day, but when your knee is killing you, it's a real grind. I was beginning to think about going into some other line of work when my girlfriend showed me a magazine article on glucosamine and chondroitin. I took the recommended dose of 1,500 milligrams for glucosamine and 1,200 milligrams for chondroitin. I did it for my girlfriend; I never thought they would do anything. It took a week before I felt any improvement, but once it started, the improvement curve got better and better. Every day it was a little better; the pain was a little less. I could do a little more. I've been taking them for two months now and I'm getting around fine at work. I'm even playing on a softball team on the weekends."

Glucosamine/chondroitin and ASU together can work wonders on your osteoarthritic joints, but they're only the beginning of the Arthritis Cure. The nine steps are an integrative treatment program that can change the course of the disease. The Arthritis Cure offers new hope to those who have been given only a few treatment options in the past. At the very least, the vast majority of patients with osteoarthritis will get *significant relief and may avoid the harmful effects of most "standard" treatments* offered by the current medical system. Results are usually seen anywhere from one to six weeks after starting to take glucosamine and chondroitin and following the rest of the program. It's important to remember, however, that just taking the supplements is not nearly as effective as following the entire nine-step plan. Glucosamine/chondroitin and ASU are powerful, but they're only the beginning of the Arthritis Cure.

The Arthritis Cure Steps

Glucosamine/chondroitin and ASU spearhead the patient-tested, nine-step Arthritis Cure plan:

1. Have a thorough consultation with a physician to get an accurate diagnosis.
2. Take glucosamine/chondroitin and ASU to repair damaged joints.
3. Improve your biomechanics to counteract stress to your joints.
4. Exercise regularly in a manner that will help and not hurt your joints.
5. Eat a healthful, joint-preserving diet, control food allergies, and take antioxidant supplements.
6. Maintain your ideal body weight. Lose weight if necessary.
7. Fight depression with counseling, SAMe, and antidepressants if necessary.
8. Use conventional medicine as necessary.
9. Maintain a positive, healthy attitude.

Millions have had great success with the Arthritis Cure for treating osteoarthritis of the knees, hips, back, neck, fingers, and other joints. It's not a cure-all, and it doesn't work for everyone, but it is undoubtedly the single most effective approach to osteoarthritis, with the least potential for harm. This program has rapidly become the gold standard for treating osteoarthritis. Let's take a look at each of the nine steps.

STEP 1 *Have a Thorough Consultation with a Physician*

A great many conditions mimic the symptoms of osteoarthritis, and many people who self-diagnose their problem do so incorrectly. As many as four in five people with chronic symptoms in a joint haven't ever actually visited a health-care professional for an accurate diagnosis and treatment.[1]

Pain in a joint can come from dozens of different sources. In some cases, a serious joint infection or even a deadly cancer can lead to chronic joint pain. Obviously, such serious causes need to be identified quickly and treated appropriately. Simply covering up the pain on your own without finding the root cause could lead to disastrous results.

Self-diagnosing the cause of chronic joint pain can lead to unnecessary pain and suffering. Bursitis, for example, causes symptoms similar to those of osteoarthritis and can last for years, but is relatively easy to cure with proper stretching and strengthening exercises. In most cases gout can be controlled if properly diagnosed and treated. Many patients live with correctable problems for years, not knowing that they don't have to. Even experienced family physicians sometimes have trouble diagnosing and treating secondary osteoarthritis; other health professionals such as chiropractors aren't well qualified to make the diagnosis. For the most accurate diagnosis, get an evaluation from a specialist physician. In general, rheumatologists, sports medicine physicians and physical medicine and rehabilitation doctors spend more time studying osteoarthritis and have more experience seeing osteoarthritis patients than other types of physicians. Orthopedic surgeons, as the name implies, spend a great deal of time and effort learning the latest in surgical care. Despite specializing in the musculoskeletal system, a surgeon may not be the best first choice for evaluating your osteoarthritis and recommending the proper *nonsurgical* care. Surgical treatment for osteoarthritis, as we'll discuss below, is often not necessary. And remember, every person has special medical concerns and not everybody responds in the same way to the same medical treatment. Always consult with your doctor before starting the

Arthritis Cure program For the latest information, side effects, and warnings concerning treatments for osteoarthritis, check my Web site at www.drtheo.com.

STEP 2 *Take Glucosamine/Chondroitin and ASU to Repair Damaged Joints*

These three disease-improving supplements are the heart of my Arthritis Cure treatment program.

So many glucosamine/chondroitin products are on the market today that it's often difficult to choose which one might be the best for you. Unfortunately, as we'll see in the next chapter, only a handful of the 200 or more available products are acceptable.

The supplements have a remarkable safety record. Hundreds of millions of doses of all three have been used worldwide without any significant problems—as long as you stick to the recommended brands.

The general dose for an adult is 1,500 mg of (active) glucosamine and 1,200 mg of chondroitin, once daily, with or without food. I'm working on a special form of chondroitin that will allow you to take only 800 mg of chondroitin per day. This will lower the cost of the supplements and decrease the size of the tablets or capsules.

For avocado soybean unsaponifiables (ASU) the dose is 300 mg (ASU or ASP), once daily, with or without food. ASU can be taken at the same time as your glucosamine/chondroitin.

All three of these supplements do not have any known interactions with other medications, so they appear to be safe when taken together. Nevertheless, if there's any concern, simply take the supplements a few hours before or after the other medications.

We have learned so much since the first edition of *The Arthritis Cure* came out in 1997. No longer do we judge the success of the supplements based just on how much or how little pain relief they provide—although the supplements have a better overall record at pain relief and improvement of function than even the most expensive prescription, anti-inflammatory drugs. Glucosamine, chondroitin, and ASU benefit the health of the joint whether or not the user experiences any pain relief! Cartilage gain or loss is painless, because cartilage itself has no nerve endings. The supplements help preserve and even rebuild the cartilage, whether or not they also relieve pain.

Let's put this in other terms. Like most people, once you start the supplements you may start experiencing pain relief quickly, possibly within just a few days, though it's much more likely to be a few weeks. Sometimes people notice improvement only after months of use. But suppose you use these supplements for a period of eight to twelve weeks and don't notice any effect? Should you stop taking them? The answer is clearly no. Long-term, carefully controlled studies indicate that after two or three years of use, even people who take the supplements and have little or no pain relief still were found to have slowed the cartilage loss in their joints. Pain is not the measure we now use to judge how well these supplements are benefiting your joints. Following your X rays over time and tracking your level of functional improvement are the best measures. The greater your function, the more you can do, whether it be walking, biking, gardening, playing sports, or any other of your usual activities.

There's another important measure of success. If the supplements are able to keep you off anti-inflammatory drugs, this alone is something to celebrate. As you'll learn, if you can avoid using anti-inflammatory drugs, you should—you could be saving your own life.

Symptoms such as pain are unrelated to what is actually going on in the joint cartilage. You can cover up painful joint symptoms by taking nonsteroidal anti-inflammatory drugs or even narcotic painkillers, but even if the pain subsides, the cartilage in the joints continues to deteriorate, perhaps even at an accelerated pace. Covering up your symptoms with pain pills without doing anything to improve your joint health makes about as much as sense as ripping the wires out of your car's dashboard if the engine warning light comes on! Pain relief, along with a program to improve joint health, is the answer.

The unlinking of symptoms to a disease process is common. Many disease-improving treatments can't be judged based on how well or poorly they control symptoms. For instance, in treating and preventing osteoporosis (bone loss), we know that it's an absolute necessity to supplement your diet with calcium, vitamin D, and perhaps magnesium if you are not getting adequate amounts in the foods you eat each day. But when they take these supplements, *people don't feel any different.* The supplements are critical to bone health and are part of the program for preventing bone loss over a long period of time, but since you can't feel bone loss or gain, you can't tell if the supplements are or are not working based on your symptoms or feelings. The same goes for your cartilage when you take glucosamine/chondroitin and ASU. Osteoarthritis is a chronic condition, and your cartilage can continue to deteriorate even if your pain disappears and your function returns to normal. By continuing to take the supplements even after your arthritis has improved or disappeared, you keep the cartilage healthy and help prevent future problems.

STEP 3   *Improve Your Biomechanics to Counteract Stress to Your Joints*

Biomechanics is the study of the mechanical forces exerted on the body by movement. Improper alignment or incorrect use of muscles, bones, tendons, ligaments, and joints can cause excessive wear and tear on the body, leading to injury. The importance of biomechanics in treating osteoarthritis can't be overstated: If you don't correct the underlying problems, you can't rid yourself of the disease.

If the wheels on a car are out of alignment, they will wear badly. You wouldn't just slap a patch on the bald spot or go to the expense of getting new tires. Instead, you fix the alignment. That's what improving biomechanics can do for your joints—fix the alignment. Many patients have enjoyed "miracle cures" by simply changing the way they walk. Whether you're a serious athlete, just a weekend dabbler, or someone who hates to exercise, you may benefit from a biomechanical evaluation, especially if you have any genetic predisposition toward osteoarthritis. An evaluation will tell you how you are using your joints, the type of stress they are subjected to, and whether you are doing anything that might contribute to the development of osteoarthritis down the line. By zeroing in on potential problem areas, you can change the way you use the joint now in order to decrease the risk of problems later. Sports medicine physicians, osteopathic manipulative medicine practitioners, some physical therapists and exercise physiologists, and neuromuscular therapists are among the many professionals who can evaluate and treat biomechanical problems.

STEP 4 *Exercise Regularly*

Regular, lifelong exercise fends off a host of health problems. It's also a great way to burn calories and lose weight. And, although we used to think that exercise caused arthritis, we now know that regular, proper exercise is an excellent means of helping to keep joints healthy. With normal joint alignment and muscle development, the idea that high-impact exercises such as running could "wear out" joints has been disproved.[2] In fact, regular exercise is strong protection against osteoarthritis.[3] When you bear down on a joint, as you do when exercising, the nutrient-rich fluid in the cartilage is squeezed out, just as if the cartilage were a soggy sponge. Then, when you release the pressure this fluid rushes back into the cartilage, both nourishing it and keeping it moist. The continual rushing in and out of fluid is critical to the health of the cartilage, not only to the matrix, but to the cartilage cells themselves. Without exercise, the cartilage becomes thin, dry, and more susceptible to damage. In addition to keeping the "cartilage sponge" in action, the proper exercises strengthen the structures around a joint, which helps to reduce the pressure the joint is subjected to.

Exercise is also a wonderful medicine for existing osteoarthritis. It keeps the nourishing fluid flowing into the afflicted joint, and reduces pressure on the joint by strengthening supporting structures. The right exercises can often reduce pain and increase mobility. And of course, exercise is essential to weight control. (See chapter 8 for more on the value of exercise.)

STEP 5 *Eat a Healthful, Joint-Preserving Diet*

What you eat (or don't eat) can affect your joints. Certain foods can encourage or discourage the joint-busting free radicals, help to increase or decrease inflammation, and stimulate cartilage repair. The healthful diet described in chapter 9 lays out a complete nutrition program for counteracting the effects of osteoarthritis while keeping your joints—and the rest of your body—healthy.

In addition to eating well, it's important to discover any food allergies or intolerances you might have that could be affecting your arthritis. I discuss this important topic more in chapter 9.

Antioxidant supplements are crucial for helping glucosamine/chondroitin and ASU work more effectively, as well for countering joint-damaging free radicals in your body. In particular, vitamin C and the mineral manganese increase the effectiveness of both glucosamine and chondroitin and have beneficial effects on joint functions. Make sure these are either included in the supplements that you buy or take them separately.

Manganese, which is important for the synthesis of cartilage components, is also an antioxidant. A deficiency of this mineral, which you need in only trace amounts, can often go unnoticed and can lead to osteoarthritis. Found in many whole foods such as nuts, beans, oatmeal, beef liver, oranges, spinach, blueberries, and raisins, manganese is usually lacking in processed foods. The Institute of Medicine says that total intake of manganese from food and supplements is safe in amounts up to 10 milligrams per day.

Vitamin C serves as an antioxidant that "recharges" other antioxidants. Because it is water-soluble, vitamin C is eliminated from the body in just a few hours (even the "time-released" kind), so taking several smaller doses throughout the day is much more effective than taking one large dose. I generally recommend taking between 60 and 500 milligrams of vitamin C per day in one to two divided doses. Even if you just take it once a day, you'll still get the benefit of vitamin C, because that's enough for your body to make the collagen you need for healthy joints and connective tissue.

STEP 6 *Maintain Your Ideal Body Weight*

Excess pounds are bad news for weight-bearing joints such as the hips and knees. Researchers have conclusively linked weight gain and obesity to osteoarthritis, specifically of the knee.[4] In a study done at Chicago's Cook County Hospital, doctors noticed that obesity was common in osteoarthritis patients, and that a large percentage of them had gained weight just before the disease hit. Fifty percent of those with osteoarthritis had been overweight for three to 10 years prior to the onset of the disease.[5]

Keeping your weight under control is a crucial part of the Arthritis Cure, for some joints must bear dozens of times the impact of your body weight during normal, everyday activities. If you gain just 10 pounds, you may be increasing the force certain joints must bear from 25 pounds up to 100 pounds! That's why staying slim is one of the most important things you can do for the life of your joints, and that's why you'll find tips for shedding excess pounds in chapter 9.

STEP 7 *Fight Depression*

It's easy to slide into depression when you can't move without pain, when everything you do seems to be a gigantic effort, and when you feel so *old* all the time. The treatment for arthritis is in you. *You* are the one who needs to take the steps to overcome this condition—not your doctor, not your partner or spouse. People with depression are less likely to be motivated to take action. Depression can worsen your pain and interfere with your recovery, so it's vital to begin smiling again as soon as possible. In chapter 10 you'll learn how to handle the psychological aspects of osteoarthritis, and how positive thinking can energize you as it sets you on the road to recovery.

STEP 8 *Use Conventional Medicine as Necessary*

In the vast majority of cases, people who follow the treatment program in the Arthritis Cure are able to avoid the side effects and dangers of arthritis drugs. In some cases, people skimp on some of the important steps detailed in the program; in others, they simply require some additional intervention, usually because they have very advanced osteoarthritis. Although drugs should be used only as a last resort, they can sometimes be the answer for particularly stubborn cases. Before you try them, learn exactly what they can and cannot offer by reading about pain pills in chapter 7.

An FDA-approved treatment for osteoarthritis of the knee (it's occasionally used for other joints as well) is a series of injections of *hyaluronans* right into the affected joint. As you recall from chapter 2, hyaluronans helped make the joint fluid thicker and more able to lubricate and absorb shock. Overall, after a series of three to five weekly injections, some patients have pain relief for up to a year. The relief is similar to what people experience from anti-inflammatory drugs, but without the side effects. Of the two major hyaluronan products on the market, Hyalgan® and Synvisc®, I prefer to use Hyalgan. Synvisc is a semisynthetic version that has been associated with severe reactions in the joints; Hyalgan doesn't have this problem and can be repeated in those patients who experienced relief from the first series of injections. Overall, about 50 percent of those who try the injections experience noticeable relief. The cost is usually covered by health insurance.

In some cases of osteoarthritis of the knee, a special brace that unloads the force on the affected side of the joint (the Generation 2 Unloader® brace) can give people tremendous relief of pain and improvement of function. The improvement is on a par with a common but radical surgical procedure called an osteotomy. This particular brace has some very good scientific evidence to support its use. In my professional experience, most of the copycat products don't work as well. The good part about using this custom-designed brace is that you can take it off. You can't undo surgery once it's been done! A careful examination and X rays are performed to see if you'd be a good candidate for the brace.

Glucosamine/chondroitin and ASU may help delay the need for surgery. Hundreds of people have canceled their appointments to have surgery for osteoarthritis, including people scheduled for joint replacements. Untold thousands have probably delayed their surgeries because of the improvements they had with the program. In many cases, delaying surgery is advisable since the skill of the surgeons, artificial joints, and surgical procedures all improve as time goes on.

Surgery may still be a final option for osteoarthritis sufferers who have little or no cartilage left (end-stage cartilage loss). In some cases, surgery can help to relieve pain, increase the joint range of motion, and help you get around more easily. Surgery can also be used to align deformed joints. Even if you are having surgery, however, you can benefit from taking glucosamine/chondroitin and ASU. The supplements can help keep you as functional as possible until the surgery takes place and can help with pre- or postsurgery rehabilitation. Glucosamine/chondroitin may also help keep an artificial joint from loosening.

The most common surgery for osteoarthritis is a simple arthroscopy, used as both a diagnostic and a therapeutic procedure. The orthopedic surgeon makes three small holes around the knee joint and uses a tiny fiber-optic video camera to look directly into the joint. The surgeon can see the condition of the cartilage and assess the integrity of the other joint structures. Loose pieces of cartilage and bone can be removed, small tears can be trimmed, and in some cases tears of the meniscus cartilage can be sewn in an attempt to repair this important structure.

A promising new procedure for areas of osteoarthritis within the joint is called microfracture. This procedure is generally performed on small areas of cartilage degeneration that are usually two centimeters or less. A sharp surgical instrument is used to punch small holes through the calcified cartilage and into the bone in an effort to release some of the bone marrow cells, induce minor bleeding, and release growth factors that can help stimulate cartilage repair. Glucosamine/

chondroitin supplements are almost always prescribed after this procedure. This technique has somewhat replaced an earlier procedure called *abrasion*, in which the surgeon simply ground down the cartilage to the bone in an attempt to form some scar tissue. Abrasion is being used less in arthroscopic surgery because we know that the scar tissue produced is inferior to normal cartilage. It doesn't absorb shock well and tends to break down within a few months to a couple of years. Patients undergoing an abrasion procedure can often feel worse or be less functional after the surgery. In fact, a recent controlled study suggests that arthroscopic knee surgery is no better than a placebo for relieving symptoms.[6]

Autologous chondrocyte implantation or ACI has gotten a lot of press over the last few years. In this procedure, the surgeon removes some of your own healthy cartilage cells from the affected joint during arthroscopic surgery. The cells are then sent off to a lab, grown and multiplied several-fold, and sent back to the surgeon. In a second surgical procedure, your own cartilage cells are placed back into the area of cartilage damage. A variety of techniques is used to attempt to keep the cells where they need to stay while the cartilage matrix attempts to heal. When successful, the new cartilage that grows is more like the original cartilage than the scar tissue that forms after an abrasion procedure. Unfortunately, ACI tends to work only in younger patients who have suffered acute trauma to the joint resulting in a well-defined area of damage to the cartilage, rather than your typical person who has osteoarthritis with cartilage erosions located in multiple areas of the joint. Another potential limitation to the use of ACI is that growing and multiplying the cells in the lab may cause them to age prematurely.[7] This might limit the long-term success of the surgical procedure.

The "end of the line" procedure for someone with severe osteoarthritis is to have a joint replacement. This procedure is most successful in the hip joint, less so in the knee. Replacements for other joints such as the elbow, shoulder, and ankle are still relative primitive. Joint replacement surgery is extremely complex and invasive and not without risk; a very small percentage of people die from complications, including blood clots, infection, or heart and lung problems. Some

120,000 hip replacement operations are performed each year in the United States. The results from a successful joint replacement can dramatically improve the quality of life in someone with severe osteoarthritis who hasn't responded to conservative therapies. Some recent evidence suggests that people who need this surgery shouldn't wait until their functional level has declined too much. The success rate for good outcomes is better in patients who have maintained some of their functional ability and are able to perform some rehabilitation exercises prior to surgery. The decision to have joint replacement surgery is up to you, however. Many people just are not psychologically ready for such a drastic step even when their doctors are encouraging the surgery. I always recommend that patients get "second opinion" consultations from specialists who are either surgeons with a reputation for being conservative, or osteoarthritis or sports medicine specialists who are not surgeons. This way, the information will not be considered biased compared to a recommendation by the operating physician alone. Most insurance companies will pay for second opinions, since they are cost-effective. Based on the second opinion, some people opt out of the surgery, at a huge cost savings for the insurer.

STEP 9 *Maintain a Positive Attitude*

Your attitude toward your condition can make a huge difference, as it does in every other aspect of life. The new medical science called psychoneuroimmunology has shown that the immune system and other parts of the body respond to negative and positive thoughts. In a landmark study, a researcher at UCLA had actors act out "happy" and "sad" scenes. When the actors were simply *pretending* to be happy, their immune systems became a little stronger, as measured by the amount of secretory immunoglobulin A. But when they pretended to be sad, their immune systems grew temporarily weaker.[8]

Staying tuned to the positive is a special kind of medicine that can be of value no matter what disease you may be facing. Here are some suggestions to help keep you on the right psychological track:

1. *Don't obsess about your condition.* Complaining and wondering "Why me?" can sap your energy and prevent you from attacking the problem head-on. Focus on your treatment, not on what the disease has done to your life. Keep thinking about how good you are going to feel soon, and how much you're going to love getting around just as you used to. The mind-body link cannot be ignored.

2. *Use guided imagery or meditation to help keep you calm and in touch with your body.* A cognitive-behavioral therapist can teach you these techniques (see chapter 10 on depression for more on this).

3. *Stay connected to friends and family.* Loneliness is a tremendous risk factor for a multitude of diseases, especially for the elderly. Those who are lonely or isolated don't respond to treatment nearly as well as those who are well connected to a spouse or life partner, family, friends, and their communities. Stay in touch with family and friends; stay involved with life. Get out as much as possible. If you can't get out, invite your friends to visit you. Even getting a pet can be helpful.

4. *Develop a sense of purpose.* People who turn adversity into a challenge have a better prognosis in the long run. If you're hurting, help others, find creative ways to do things you otherwise wouldn't be able to, and look for a beneficial message in your condition. Situations that most people think are hopeless often lead to good.

The positive is always out there, waiting to be seen and used.

—6—

CHOOSING AND USING ARTHRITIS SUPPLEMENTS

What are the most effective doses?

How can you choose quality supplements?

What supplement forms are available?

What safety issues should you understand?

Which products are the best?

My mission in developing the arthritis cure was to give people a safer, more effective alternative for treating osteoarthritis. Enlightening the public and the medical community on the benefits of glucosamine and chondroitin were keys to this goal. Now that this goal is well under way, my new mission is to steer people toward quality supplements, the kinds that are actually effective, while alerting people to fraudulent and substandard products. Poor-quality products keep people from benefiting fully from the program and harm the reputation of this great treatment.

I have personally investigated and paid for lab analyses of several of the joint-health products currently on the market. Other organizations have done the same. Based on this information, I feel confident that the recommendations I make later in this chapter—of both high-quality products and products to avoid—have a solid basis in fact, not advertising hype.

The Right Dose for You

How large a dose do you need to get the benefits of glucosamine/ chondroitin and ASU? Here's what I usually recommend:

- Glucosamine: 1,500 mg glucosamine HCl or 1,884 mg glucosamine sulfate, taken once daily or divided into two equal doses.
- Chondroitin: 800 to 1,200 mg, taken once daily or divided into two equal doses.
- ASU: 300 mg, taken once daily

Let's look more closely at the evidence for these doses and the best way to make sure you're getting the full dose of an effective, high-quality supplement.

Glucosamine Dose

Nearly every controlled study of glucosamine uses the equivalent of 1,500 mg of glucosamine hydrochloride (HCl) or 1,884 mg of glucosamine sulfate (SO_4) as the effective treatment dose. What's the difference? Glucosamine alone is unstable; it likes to break apart or bind with something else. To make it stable, glucosamine is attached to other molecules. The two most common ones are hydrochloride (HCl) or the larger and heavier molecule *sulfate*. Because of the weight difference, glucosamine attached to sulfate is heavier than glucosamine attached to hydrochloride. Therefore, to get the same amount of free glucosamine, one would need to take 1,884 mg of glucosamine sulfate to get the same amount of glucosamine as in 1,500 mg of glucosamine HCl. This is not where the story ends, however. Glucosamine sulfate, though more stable than glucosamine alone, can turn brown or become less potent unless it is further stabilized by mixing it with additional salts, either sodium chloride (NaCl, or table salt) or potassium chloride (KCl).

In the first step of the process, after adding the sulfate component, you would need to take 1,884 mg of glucosamine sulfate to get 1,500 mg of glucosamine HCl, because the *sulfate* portion takes up more space and adds weight. But you can't buy glucosamine sulfate unless it is stabilized with salt. The legitimate products on the market (from perhaps only 5 to 10 percent of the companies selling it—I'll discuss this more below) adjust for this process. For example, when they say, "Three capsules provide 1,500 mg of glucosamine sulfate," they're really packaging over 2,000 mg of the stabilized salt form in order to assure that they're delivering the equivalent of 1,500 mg of glucosamine HCl.

Unfortunately, the amounts of the salts added can vary widely in most (but not all) glucosamine sulfate products. If the companies don't tell you exactly how much salt is used to stabilize the glucosamine sulfate, you really don't know the *glucosamine HCl* equivalents you're getting. In many cases, you'll need to take *more* than 2,500 mg of salt-stabilized glucosamine sulfate to get 1,500 of glucosamine HCl—but you wouldn't know this unless you had the laboratory analysis of the product. Because many manufacturers skimp on the glucosamine sulfate by adding more salt, you're not getting the benefit of the right dose and you might be getting unhealthy doses of sodium or potassium from some low-quality brands. I'm sure this is why some people have told me their blood pressure went up after they used certain brands.

Even though some supplement manufacturers state on the label that their products are "laboratory tested" or "guaranteed pure," in reality, they may not be. In many cases, the companies are making these claims not based on testing performed on their finished product, but on a document called a certificate of analysis they received from the bulk, raw material supplier. This document is supposed to be a laboratory analysis of the bulk material, but sadly, these documents are sometimes not accurate or are even fabricated, especially in products coming from overseas. Some raw material suppliers are even more underhanded—they may put some of the pure active ingredient on the surface of a large container, but the material below the surface might be something different, such as plain sugar, which is much, much cheaper than good-quality glucosamine.

Why would a raw material supplier stoop to such levels? Profit. Many of these suppliers are based in foreign countries and cannot be sued or prosecuted in the United States if they're caught selling substandard product. They know that the worst that usually happens is that the manufacturer finds out and rejects the material. If the raw material companies sell this cheap, inferior product to U.S. manufacturers, and if the U.S. manufacturers don't properly test the material prior to using it, then perhaps no one will know that the end product is simply a placebo, or worse—it might contain something that is not safe. Unscrupulous bulk suppliers get away with inferior products or skimping on quality control and testing because they know a lot of supplement manufacturers are just looking to buy the cheapest product so they can sell it cheaply to the consumer or realize a higher profit.

Even when supplement manufacturers make certain to buy only high-quality raw materials, they don't always make the proper adjustment to the dose to be sure the supplement contains the right amount of glucosamine base. Why? In my opinion, for any one or more of three possible reasons: The manufacturers don't understand this basic principle of chemistry (in which case they have no right producing products for human consumption); they rely solely on the analysis provided by the supplier of the bulk material ingredients (another faux pas, since these can be inaccurate and it violates the voluntary rules of good manufacturing practices—I'll discuss those below); or they're simply greedy for higher profits. No matter what the reason, the result is unacceptable. No product that you consume for your health should be produced with any shortcuts in quality.

Supplement manufacturers still need to test their product after it is manufactured and put on the shelf for sale. A lot can go wrong in processing: improper product labeling and storage, failure to properly clean mixing and processing equipment, accidental addition of unwanted materials, and much more. Only tests performed *after* processing can verify if the product meets quality standards. The label can list 1,500 mg of glucosamine, but this is often not exactly what's in the bottle. Unless companies are testing every single batch of every product, they really don't know for sure what they're selling. This explains why I would avoid over 90 percent of the products on the market.

Taking subpotent products, ones that don't use quality ingredients, or products that are not manufactured with the proper controls, is not simply a waste of time and money. Because these supplements are disease modifying, if you take imposters, you are not getting the wonderful benefits of their action. Your cartilage is probably degenerating unnecessarily and you may have to use dangerous anti-inflammatory drugs and pain relievers, or even have unnecessary surgery. This, to my mind, is a tragedy. It is unacceptable ethically and morally, it's limiting the acceptance of a valid treatment in the medical community, and it's causing people to suffer needlessly. There's no need to experiment with your health when there are better, safer choices. Almost every time someone writes to tell me that he or she had no success with a particular product, it's because they have been taking a fraudulent product. When I suggest switching to a reputable brand, the person finally gets the benefits of the supplements.

An independent analysis published in 2002 in a leading rheumatology journal evaluated 15 different glucosamine-containing products. The results were astounding. The analysis revealed that almost all products failed to supply the recommended dose of glucosamine. Only *one* out of 15 products tested contained the required amount of 90 to 110 percent of label claim.[1]

Chondroitin Dose

The issues related to quality and proper dosing of chondroitin are actually even more complex than for glucosamine. It's important to understand some of these issues to help choose a quality brand that will actually do something to improve the condition of your joints. You certainly don't want to spend your money on a product that appears to be acceptable and may even help relieve your pain, but is not doing its main function, which is improving the health of your joints.

Largely due to more complex processing steps, chondroitin sulfate per gram is approximately four to eight times more expensive than glucosamine. As a result, those companies more interested in profit than quality may try to skimp on chondroitin by:

- providing less than is listed on the label
- using dosages lower than those supported in the research
- substituting cheaper, less active, or inactive substances for chondroitin
- obtaining chondroitin from companies that don't follow the strictest quality standards in processing

The usual recommended dose for chondroitin is 1,200 mg daily—that's the dose used in studies that have shown benefit in reducing pain and increasing function. Taking it once a day is just as effective as dividing the dose in thirds and taking it three times a day.[2] Since the original publication of *The Arthritis Cure,* there have been a number of new studies published on the oral use of chondroitin. Several studies, including the powerful, two-year, disease-modifying study for osteoarthritis that showed chondroitin could halt loss of cartilage from osteoarthritis, have shown that just 800 mg is effective.[3] So, if the proper kind of chondroitin is used, 800 mg per day is an acceptable treatment dose. Taking 1,200 mg daily or even more is perfectly safe, but there's no evidence to show that taking a larger dose than that will help you more. To be sure you're really getting the amount of chondroitin you need, choose a high-quality product from a reputable manufacturer.

Avocado-Soy Unsaponifiables (ASU) Dose

When avocado soy unsaponifiables (ASU) become widely available as a supplement, a rash of poor-quality copycat products will undoubtedly hit the market soon after the public becomes aware of how well this supplement works. Many supplement companies simply wait for the next big thing to come along, even if it has no scientific merit. One of the ways I identify reputable companies is to look at how quickly they jump on the bandwagon versus how careful they are in investigating the validity of a product or intervention.

Creating a quality ASU or avocado soy phytosterols (ASP) product is even more complicated than making glucosamine or chondroitin.

There are multiple active ingredients in ASU that need very careful handling to be purified and stabilized. I think it highly likely that some unscrupulous companies will simply sell supplements containing avocado and soy oils, and not the active ASU ingredients in the quantities known to benefit the joints. Avocado and soy oils do not contain the same active components, in the same quantities, as the highly processed, purified, and concentrated ingredients in the valid products. As the new products become available, I'll be investigating them very carefully. The information will be available to everyone on my Web site at www.drtheo.com. I'll update it frequently as new products come onto the market.

The Safety of the Supplements

Glucosamine/chondroitin have an outstanding safety record. Cases of adverse reactions, overdoses, and other problems with these supplements are almost nonexistent. The few safety concerns about them turn out to be more myth than fact.

Glucosamine and diabetes: All worked up over nothing.   Years ago, based on some small animal studies that utilized very high-dose glucosamine given intravenously, I raised the theoretical possibility that glucosamine could increase blood sugar. Until we had controlled research to suggest otherwise, my recommendation was that people with diabetes should monitor their blood sugar closely when taking glucosamine. The research on animals was never very convincing, however, because the doses were so much higher than the comparative dose a human would take. Thousands of times higher, in fact. For that reason, diabetes was never a contraindication to using glucosamine, and none of my patients with diabetes ever had a problem with the supplement. Even so, a rumor got started that glucosamine adversely affects blood sugar. Perhaps this was because of the similarity of the words "glucosamine" and "glucose." Glucosamine and glucose are in reality very different and follow different pathways in the body once ingested. Even if they were equal, however, the daily dose of

1.5 grams is less glucose than you would find in a single grape or an ounce of a sugary soft drink—an amount that is very unlikely to have an effect on a person with diabetes.

Studies on humans investigating this possible link have concluded that this is a nonissue. In a randomized, double-blind, placebo-controlled trial using a combination of 1,500 mg of glucosamine and 1,200 mg of chondroitin, 28 elderly patients with stable Type 2 (adult-onset) diabetes received the supplements; 12 received a placebo. After 90 days of treatment, there was no difference between the groups in HbA1c, a long-term marker of blood glucose and diabetes control.[4] Long-term evidence against glucosamine causing diabetes was found in a large, three-year, placebo-controlled glucosamine study in 2001. The participants using glucosamine actually had a slightly *lower* fasting glucose level compared with those taking the placebo.[5]

An important factor in controlling (and preventing) insulin resistance and Type 2 diabetes is exercise. People hampered by arthritis generally don't exercise enough—they are in pain and often become sedentary. This lack of activity can contribute to obesity, insulin resistance, and diabetes. People with diabetes are much more likely to develop kidney diseases—and the medicines typically used for osteoarthritis (acetaminophen and anti-inflammatories) are very toxic to the kidneys. It stands to reason that the supplements, which have not shown any adverse effects on kidney function, are a much better choice for people with diabetes.

Chondroitin and mad cow disease (BSE).   Some critics of dietary supplements, who appear to have felt especially threatened by the success of chondroitin, tried to create rumors about the theoretical possibility of a connection between mad cow disease and chondroitin obtained from bovine (cow) sources.

The factual information to support these rumors never materialized and the FDA declared that there should be little or no concern. (We should be much more concerned about salmonella or E. coli bacterial infections in our meat and dairy supply. In 2001, about 71,000 cases of E. coli infection occurred the United States alone.) The odds against a chondroitin or glucosamine product containing bacteria are astronomical. The processing steps would destroy all bacteria even if contaminated raw material was inadvertantly used as a source, and to my knowledge no product has ever tested positive for bacteria.

Infection from a prion, the agent that causes mad cow disease, is also extremely unlikely if not impossible. For well over a decade, the FDA has had very severe regulations and restrictions on imports into the United States of food products and supplements originating from cattle. All foods, dietary supplements, and pharmaceutical products derived from cattle have had safeguards to prevent any BSE from entering the United States. This program has been an amazing success. Hundreds of millions of servings of food and supplements derived from cattle have been consumed by U.S. citizens since the concern over BSE first arose, and not a single case of BSE-tainted food or supplements has been uncovered. No cases of BSE have originated and materialized in the United States.

The quality control processes used by manufacturers further limit the risk of BSE. Only cows from certified non-BSE countries are used in the manufacturing process. Chondroitin is extracted from parts of the cow with a lot of cartilage, such as the trachea. The brain and spinal cord, which can transmit BSE, are not used. The manufacturing process requires enzymatic digestion of proteins—and because the prion that causes BSE is actually a fragment of protein, it should be destroyed.

Of course, if you have any concerns at all, consider using chondroitin produced entirely in the United States. In any event, the risk is highly theoretical. Despite hundreds of millions of doses over many years no one has ever developed BSE from consuming chondroitin. The daily real-world concern is that on average, NSAIDs lead to over 45 deaths per day, every day of the year.

Glucosamine and shellfish allergies.   Thousands of people in the United States have severe and sometimes life-threatening allergies to shellfish products. (An allergy to shellfish, by the way, is not the same as the food poisoning that can result from eating poorly handled shellfish!) People who are truly allergic to shellfish react to a protein in the "meat" portion of the shellfish. The vast majority of glucosamine products are derived from the shells of shrimp, lobster, and crabs, but the protein isn't found in the shells. It is possible, however, especially with lower quality manufacturers, that tiny bits of protein fragments from the meat are retained in the finished glucosamine product. In this rare case, it is then possible that a person with a severe allergy to shell-fish could suffer a reaction from taking glucosamine. To date, I have not heard any reports of a life-threatening allergy from taking glu-cosamine, but I have heard of a few isolated cases of people with severe shellfish allergies who developed a self-limited rash after consuming glucosamine.

If you have a known allergy to shellfish, don't experiment with glu-cosamine unless specifically instructed to do so by your physician. Chondroitin and ASU products are not derived from shellfish. These should be considered alternatives to glucosamine containing products in people allergic to shellfish.

Another viable option is a glucosamine product called Regena-sure®. This is a vegetarian form of very pure glucosamine hydrochlo-ride that is created from a renewable resource and not from shellfish. Products made exclusively with this form of glucosamine are not required to carry a shellfish warning label. Regenasure® is also a good option for people who do not eat shellfish products for religious or personal reasons.

Choosing the Best Forms

Glucosamine/chondroitin have become so popular that they are now available in many different forms in addition to the standard tablets. Some of these products are worthwhile for their extra convenience, but most will do more to lighten your wallet than help your joints.

Be wary of products that to claim to be "long-acting," "timed-released," or "controlled-delivery." All glucosamine/chondroitin and ASU products are long-acting. They need to be taken just once a day. To make these products even more "long-acting" the manufac-turer would have to change their structure or their delivery system. In the case of glucosamine, there's some evidence that this makes the supplement less active or even inactive. Because some pain relievers are sold in time-released or controlled-delivery forms that really do work better, you might be fooled into thinking that the same is true for glucosamine. Don't fall for this marketing gimmick. You actually want the glucosamine to be released as quickly as possible. After you swallow glucosamine, about 85 to 90 percent of it is absorbed into the bloodstream. The blood vessels bring glucosamine into the joint fluid by exchange through the joint capsule. The more glucosamine that is delivered to the bloodstream, the higher the concentration that will appear in the joint fluid. Once glucosamine enters the joint fluid, it bathes the chondrocytes (cartilage cells). We know that a certain minimum concentration of glucosamine is needed for the chondrocytes to benefit. Trickling glucosamine slowly into the bloodstream means the chondrocytes are exposed to very low concentrations below the minimum threshold for any effect.

A good analogy is knocking on a neighbor's door to get his or her attention. You have to give one or two loud knocks for your neighbor to hear you. Tapping on the door very softly for a long period of time won't do the job. Your knocks won't be answered because they won't be heard.

Chondroitin and ASU are also extremely long-acting, so marketing controlled-delivery or timed-release formulas for these supplements is even more foolish.

Don't be fooled by labels that claim double or triple strength. This issue is a little confusing. For most of the combination glucosamine/chondroitin products on the market, taking enough of the product (usually the amount recommended on the label) should provide you with the recommended dosages of 1,500 mg of glucosamine and 1,200 mg of chondroitin (or 800 mg chondroitin if you're using the new form).

Manufacturers use the terms "double-strength" or "triple-strength" to indicate that you need to take fewer tablets (or capsules, caplets, or softgels) to achieve the proper dose. This is not because the products are more concentrated or potent, but because they add more glucosamine and chondroitin, making the capsule or tablet larger.

A simple way to avoid confusion is to mentally replace the word "strength" with the word "size." A double-strength tablet is simply twice the size of a single strength. Triple-strength is about three times the size.

If you have difficulty swallowing large tablets, then choose a single-strength or double-strength. If you don't mind large tablets and simply want to take the minimum number of pills, choose a triple-strength product. And remember, even if you're taking four or six single-strength tablets, you can take them all at once with or without food.

Some people have difficulty swallowing pills and supplements of any sort. A good way to get the pills down is to put a small amount of fluid (something that has some thickness to it such as milk or juice) in your mouth, then put the supplements in your mouth, sip a little more of the drink, and take one big swallow. All of the tablets and fluid should go down at once. Some people find that if they have something to eat afterward, the tablets are less likely to get stuck in the esophagus (food tube). If you have difficulty swallowing, tell your doctor. There are many medical conditions that may cause this symptom.

Be cautious of the claims on liquid glucosamine/chondroitin products. The companies that make them claim pricey liquid supplements are better than tablets, capsules, or powders because they are absorbed better into the body. There's no evidence for this. There's no problem absorbing glucosamine and chondroitin tablets, powders, caplets or capsules; all the good-quality products dissolve easily and well.

It's possible that absorption is *lower* in liquid products. We know that stomach acid is important for proper absorption of glucosamine. The liquid products could dilute this acid, interfering with absorption. When people swallow capsules or tablets, they usually just drink small amounts of liquid, compared to the 8, 10, or 12 ounces with liquid products. Furthermore, even when the liquid product is in a lower volume, people drink a lot of fluids to drown the (usually) poor taste.

There are some questions and concerns about stability of liquid products containing glucosamine sulfate. Stabilizing glucosamine with salts is critical to maintain potency, but what happens when you put salt in a liquid? The salt usually dissolves.

If you decide to use a liquid product, look for one that contains glucosamine hydrochloride—it appears to be a better choice for stability. Most liquid products that have attempted to add chondroitin have been plagued with problems concerning poor taste or smell. This problem has been remedied by a company that is found a way to process the chondroitin without any chemical solvents. Optaflex® chondroitin is the only solvent-free chondroitin currently on the market. It readily dissolves in liquid, appears to be stable, and has virtually no taste when added even to plain water.

The final concern over liquid products relates to personal preference. People often grow tired of drinking the same formula day in and day out. Since you should consider using glucosamine and chondroitin for the long term to get the maximum benefits on disease modification, you'll want to choose a product that you'd be willing to take on a consistent basis.

Be cautious of the word **complex** *in glucosamine/chondroitin products.* It generally means that other substances have been added. When done appropriately with the right additional supplements, this can help. For instance, the mineral manganese (in doses below 11 mg per day) and vitamin C are known to benefit cartilage and are useful additions to a joint-health supplement.

Unfortunately, the word complex in some products might be a signal to you that the manufacturer has diluted the glucosamine with other components, such as N-acetylglucosamine (NAG). Mixing glucosamine hydrochloride and glucosamine sulfate can result in a reduced yield of glucosamine base delivered in the product, because of the need to stabilize the sulfate form with additional salts.

The term "chondroitin complex" usually portends an ominous situation. Chondroitin is an expensive supplement. Some companies try to dilute it in any manner they can get away with to reduce the cost of manufacturing and squeeze out more profit. MSM, hydrolyzed collagen, chicken cartilage, and related substances are *not* chondroitin. By no stretch of imagination could they possibly substitute for chondroitin in a joint-health supplement, yet some companies purposely try to confuse you by adding these other components to products with such low doses of chondroitin that they can't have any benefit.

The sure sign that a product is being diluted is when the chondroitin sulfate content is not listed alone on the supplement and is instead added to a list of two or more items. So, instead of seeing only *chondroitin sulfate 1,200 mg* on the label, you might see something like this:

Chondroitin Sulfate complex 1,200 mg
   MSM
   Hydrolyzed collagen
   Chondroitin sulfate

In this case, the product may actually contain only 50 or 100 mg of chondroitin sulfate—there's no way to know exactly how much. MSM and hydrolyzed collagen are very cheap products, so there is a profit incentive to use these instead of the relatively expensive chondroitin sulfate.

Supplement manufacturers have made a number of false or misleading claims about substances that are said to be similar to chondroitin. Green-lipped mussel, sea cucumber, velvet deer antler, MSM, hydrolyzed collagen, gelatin, CMO or CM, chicken cartilage, and shark cartilage are all sold under this false promise. None of these products have substantial evidence and certainly none can claim that they can improve the disease itself.

Avoid topical forms.   Glucosamine and chondroitin applied topically (rubbed on) to the skin appear to be completely useless and a waste of money. Some companies have tried to capitalize on the popularity and name recognition of glucosamine and chondroitin by putting these oral treatments for osteoarthritis into a topical or "rub-on" cream or lotion. There is no theoretical basis for their use as a topical agent and no research to date that is of any value. Not only is it difficult or impossible to get molecules of glucosamine and chondroitin to penetrate the skin, but if you could, the concentration would likely be too low to have any physiologic effect. Basically, using topical glucosamine and chondroitin makes as much sense for treating your osteoarthritis as resting your head on a dictionary to try to improve your vocabulary.

One company sponsored a study in an effort to cite for advertising purposes. Unfortunately the study was so poorly performed that the conclusions were completely invalid and useless. Even though it was eventually published in a rheumatology journal, the study is so obviously flawed that it isn't taken seriously.

I have spoken with representatives from some companies that make topical glucosamine and chondroitin products. Each person I spoke with freely admitted that they did not believe these supplements were active when applied on the skin. They are simply playing off the public awareness of these supplements to raise the price for their products. Another indication that something is fishy is that most companies list these ingredients as "skin conditioners," and not active treatments for the pain of osteoarthritis. In this way, they're trying to sell the products as cosmetics, which have more lenient labeling and advertising guidelines compared to dietary supplements.

Use caution when a product claims that it offers a money-back guarantee.   Some of these products had the lowest content of active ingredients in independent testing. Some companies will make their products so cheaply that they know they can still make money, even if a significant percentage of their clientele returns the product for a refund. Some companies that use mail order, Web sites, or direct sales can make a profit just on the shipping and handling charges alone, even if you return the product for a refund of the product purchase price.

Be cautious of claims that something is better than glucosamine or chondroitin.   With the exception of ASU, there is nothing you can take by mouth, rub on, or inject that even comes close to glucosamine and chondroitin. In terms of effectiveness at reducing pain and increasing function and having an unmatched safety profile, these supplements have been helping people overcome osteoarthritis for years. SAMe also has benefits for treating osteoarthritis (and depression), but it is not as effective as the other three.

Occasionally companies spend a fortune on advertising to try to convince you that their study "proves" the superiority of their exclusive product to glucosamine and chondroitin. Don't believe it for a minute. In every case I've investigated so far, the "research" they cite or have performed on their product is so biased, poorly designed, or uses such a small sample that it does not provide credible evidence for *any* claims. Furthermore, such research should be reviewed and evaluated by someone who is not associated with the company, such as a peer-reviewed specialty medical journal, preferably in the area of rheumatology. More often, however, the company sponsors research only to use it directly in advertising—they won't allow it to be objectively scrutinized. By comparison, the evidence for glucosamine, chondroitin, and ASU is not only substantial, but when independent medical groups review it, they find that the supplements are the best-studied and most effective treatments available.

If some credible evidence comes out for a new product, you can be sure I'll be there to explain the results and make the proper recommendations.

Avoid Store Brands

It sure is tempting. You're at the store looking to buy a joint health supplement. Next to the name brand you've been taking for a few months is a store or generic-looking brand. It says on the label "compare to [your brand]" and even has the same color scheme and appearance. At about half the price, you think, it's hard to pass up. Think again. I get free products like this all of the time. I'd like to give them to my dog, but I care too much for him. I certainly wouldn't use them myself. I usually end up just tossing them out. Generic-looking brands and store brands are perfectly fine for many products: paper towels, laundry detergent, shampoo. They're even fine for over-the-counter drugs, because those products are regulated by the Food and Drug Administration (FDA) and must be exactly the same as their name brand counterpart. Dietary supplements, however, are not as strictly regulated. There is no government regulation to ensure that store-brand supplements are equivalent to the brand-name products or to the products that have been used in clinical research. Ask yourself, "Why am I buying this supplement?" Clearly, it's something you take for your health. It's also something you take by mouth, that gets absorbed into your body, circulates in your blood, reaches your joints, and then acts on the cartilage cells in the intended manner. Can you trust that a product will do this just because it has the words *glucosamine* and *chondroitin* listed on the label? No.

There's no such thing as a "generic" dietary supplement—there are only good-quality or poorer quality products. You may not be getting *any* active ingredient in a "generic-looking" supplement. Consider this when you're thinking of saving a few dollars on a product. Remember, you're not buying a car wax, you're buying something you put in your mouth and swallow for your health.

It is often a surprise to the consumer when they learn that the quality control practices and testing of supplements can sometimes cost *more* than the actual materials used in the supplements. So, if you combined a company's desire to simply buy the very cheapest material possible with the desire to bypass or skip some of the quality-control procedures, you have a recipe for a poor-quality product. It doesn't matter how cheap the product is—you're not getting a bargain if the product is ineffective.

Choosing Good Products

Product quality remains as the most important barrier in using glu-cosamine/chondroitin and ASU supplements for joint health. How can you know if you're buying a top-quality product? You have three resources:

- Buy products from companies that follow good manufacturing practices (GMP).
- Buy products that have also been tested and recommended by independent laboratories.
- Check my Web site at www.drtheo.com for a continuously updated list of products that meet my high standards.

Critics of dietary supplements point out that they are not regulated by the FDA. That's not quite true. Dietary supplements have been regulated as *foods* since the original Food, Drug and Cosmetic Act of 1938. This did not change with the passage of the Dietary Supplement Health and Education Act (DSHEA) in 1994. The FDA frequently wields its power to seize or ban supplements it believes are unsafe.

Provisions in DSHEA call for the development of manufacturing standards as well as tracking systems for problems related to dietary supplements. The tracking system, called the Adverse Event Reporting System or AERS, is in place. In addition, standardized good manufacturing practices (GMPs) have been published.

GMPs are currently voluntary, but quality supplement manufacturers have been using them in an effort to stand apart from those companies that do not voluntarily participate. Among other provisions, the GMPs spell out exactly how companies should receive and handle raw materials, produce supplements, check for safety, and track problems related to processing. Many of the best companies are hoping that the FDA will eventually make GMPs mandatory. Too many supplement companies don't follow GMPs and are giving the entire industry a bad reputation.

Until or unless the FDA decides to make GMPs mandatory for supplement manufacturers, compliance can be monitored and graded by third-party audits to help assure the public that the manufacturer is indeed complying with these guidelines. On the advertising front, the Federal Trade Commission (FTC) is involved with regulating advertising claims for all products, including dietary supplements.

Several independent organizations have tested products containing glucosamine and chondroitin. I have also done my own independent testing of consumer products—in fact, my study is so far the largest done by independent testing.

I purchased well over a hundred samples of glucosamine and chondroitin products and had them independently tested at a national laboratory that specializes in this area. I didn't just pick products I thought would fail. I also picked products that I suspected were of very high quality, based on their good manufacturing practices and the good clinical responses noted from my patients. I was amazed at the results.

Most of the products I *suspected* would test well did so. But overall, almost 80 percent of the samples I had tested *failed* to meet their label claims. What the company had printed on the label was not at all what was actually in the product. It didn't matter what kind of promises or quality statements were printed on the labels of the failed products.

Two of the larger selling brands tested extremely poorly. One brand averaged only about 1 percent of the label claim for chondroitin in 12 out of 14 different batches (lots) tested. The label said 400 mg chondroitin per tablet, but the tablets in these 12 lots only contained 4.4 milligrams each. The other brand failed in both glucosamine and chondroitin content. I had later learned that one of the major store chains was using the same manufacturer and material.

Four brands so far meet my stringent requirements for quality and potency; others are still being evaluated. New products that pass will be posted at www.drtheo.com. The four that have passed so far include three combination glucosamine/chondroitin products and one glucosamine-alone product.

- Osteo Bi-Flex® (Rexall)
- Cosamin DS (Nutramax Labs)
- TripleFlex® (NatureMade)
- Dona® (glucosamine alone, Rotta Pharmaceuticals)

My patients have had excellent results with these products. If you decide to choose them, be sure to buy exactly what I've written above. Some manufacturers have tried to confuse consumers with similar-sounding brand names or claim equivalency when they really shouldn't. An official "Dr. Theo" product line will appear in 2004. It will include a vegetarian and kosher option for joint health and combination products. My goal for these products is to provide the finest possible quality.

My testing results are not without corroboration. An evaluation of 32 products containing chondroitin sulfate was performed and published in the *Journal of the American Nutraceutical Association* in 2000.[6] Only five out of 32 products met label claims (that is, had in them what they said on the label). That means 84 percent *failed* to meet label claim, similar to my evaluation. In this study (which, of course did not evaluate all products on the market), products that cost less than $1 per daily dose of 1,200 mg chondroitin failed badly—they had less than 10 percent of the label claim. In other words, even though their label may have shown 1,200 mg, they actually had less than 120 mg, a dose known *not* to be effective. Interestingly, the four most expensive products in the study also failed, indicating that high cost is not a reliable indicator of quality. Very low cost was, however, a reliable indicator for identifying a poor-quality product.

Consumer Reports, in their January 2002 issue,[7] also listed their testing results of 12 brands of glucosamine and chondroitin products. Of the 12 combination products, three *failed* testing. *Consumer Reports* was the only group that listed the product failures along with the passing products. I admire their courage in doing so. *Consumer Reports*, as a large and very well-regarded organization famed for its fairness and objectivity, has no need to fear naming poor products. Based on their independent lab tests, *Consumer Reports* failed these products:

- Now Double Strength Glucosamine & Chondroitin (Now Foods)
- ArthxDS Glucosamine Chondroitin (Pecos Pharmaceuticals)
- Solgar Extra Strength Glucosamine Chondroitin Complex

One of the three chondroitin-only products also failed:

- Now Chondroitin Sulfate

And one chondroitin-only product recommended too low a dosage:

- Twinlab CSA

Consumer Labs, another independent testing organization, reported test results on combination glucosamine/chondroitin products in March 2000. Almost half (6 out of 13) of the combination products failed the testing. Testing also revealed failures for both of the chondroitin-only products they examined.

An independent analysis, published in the prestigious *Journal of Rheumatology*, evaluated 15 different glucosamine-containing products. The study revealed only *one* out of 15 products tested contained the required amount of 90 to 110 percent of the label claim. That translates into a 93 percent failure rate.[8] The passing product had 108 percent of its claim on the label, but the others averaged below 56 percent. The lowest had only 41 percent of what it claimed.

There are several third-party organizations that provide "stamps of approval" for supplement manufacturers to help ensure they are creating safe, high-quality supplements. This is certainly an evolving area, but some of the many programs include:

- USP-DSVP, the United States pharmacopoeia dietary supplement verification program
- NSF, an international dietary supplements certification program
- NNFA, the National Natural Foods Association, an industry group
- Good Housekeeping Seal of Approval
- Consumer Labs, a for-profit company that sells co-branding opportunities

In my view, the USP-DSVP is the most stringent of the programs, paying careful attention to all the major steps in the manufacture of dietary supplements. I don't believe that the other programs, as of this writing, are stringent enough in their offerings to guarantee quality, though they are likely better than no certification at all. The only exception in my opinion is Consumer Labs. In their initial assessment of joint health products, they gave a pass to products even when the chondroitin component could have failed in two out of three tests. I do not feel this is acceptable.

If you're in doubt about a product, please check my Web site. I will continue to recommend products only from reputable companies that implement GMPs *and* undergo independent testing after production. Glucosamine, chondroitin, and ASU have become so important for millions of people that we should not leave quality control to chance.

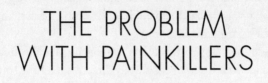

—7—
THE PROBLEM
WITH PAINKILLERS

What kind of painkillers are used to
treat osteoarthritis?

What is acetaminophen?

What are the side effects and risks
of acetaminophen?

What is a nonsteroidal anti-inflammatory
drug (NSAID)?

How do NSAIDs work?

What is a COX-2 inhibitor NSAID?

Which NSAIDs are best for osteoarthritis?

What are the side effects and risks of
using NSAIDS?

Can NSAIDs actually make osteoarthritis worse?

Can NSAIDs be combined with
glucosamine/chondroitin and ASU therapy?

Are there natural replacements for NSAIDs?

What other pain relievers are used
for osteoarthritis?

You've heard this tag line over and over: for treatment of the pain of osteoarthritis. It's part of every ad for over-the-counter and prescription painkillers. What the ads don't say is anything about treating the source of the pain—nothing about joint health, nothing about improving the disease, nothing about slowing cartilage loss. These drugs help the pain but leave the underlying disease untouched—or even make it worse.

Glucosamine/chondroitin, along with ASU, are the treatment of first choice for your osteoarthritis. They directly target the source of the problem, instead of simply masking the symptoms. They are disease-modifying treatments, not just symptom-modifying treatments. And in carefully controlled clinical trials, they have been shown to improve pain and function in osteoarthritis just as well as the most commonly used pain relievers, but without the potentially serious effects these drugs can have.

I feel it is only a matter of time before it will be considered medical malpractice to prescribe drugs to osteoarthritis patients without also trying to improve their condition with the supplements and other steps outlined in this book.

Even so, glucosamine/chondroitin and ASU take time to work, and not everyone responds the same way. There well may be times when painkillers are a necessary temporary addition to the Arthritis Cure. In fact, I use painkillers in my practice for the small number of patients who need additional relief.

If you decide to use painkillers, you can still continue to take glucosamine/chondroitin and ASU. The supplements will continue to work with the medication, and vice versa—the supplements won't affect how well the painkillers work. In fact, if you use painkilling anti-inflammatory drugs, it's even more important to use the supplements as well to help counteract the additional damage these drugs can do to your joints. Over time, the supplements can also save you money by allowing you to reduce the dose and possibly even eliminate the drugs altogether.

Before swallowing any medication, it's important that you understand just what its supposed to do—and what its side effects may do to you.

In recent years we've learned a lot about the best ways to use painkillers, and we've seen the arrival of some new pain medications. We've also learned a great deal about the potential dangers and downside to these drugs.

THESE SUPPLEMENTS ARE SAFE

In head-to-head comparisons, not only are glucosamine/chondroitin and ASU more effective than NSAIDs for long-term use, they're far safer. As shown by dozens of carefully controlled clinical studies, not a single death worldwide has been attributed to these supplements after hundreds of millions of doses over many years. By comparison, at any given time, more than 13 million Americans are taking an anti-inflammatory drug—and these drugs lead to some 16,500 deaths and 103,000 hospitalizations every year.[1]

Old and New Pain Medications

Although there are numerous pain drugs with exotic-sounding names, those prescribed for osteoarthritis generally fall into one of two categories:

- acetaminophen
- nonsteroidal anti-inflammatory drugs (NSAIDs)

You're undoubtedly familiar with acetaminophen. It's sold over-the-counter under brand names such as Tylenol® Datril®, and Liquiprin® in addition to generic versions. And you've almost certainly already taken an over-the-counter nonsteroidal anti-inflammatory drug, or NSAID (pronounced EN-sade). These are drugs such as aspirin, ibuprofen (such as Advil® and Motrin®), or naproxen (such as Aleve® and Naprosyn®). COX-2 inhibitors, also known as COX-2 NSAIDs, are newer versions of NSAIDs. These prescription drugs are heavily advertised under the brand names Vioxx®, Celebrex®, and Bextra®.

There are major differences between acetaminophen and the NSAIDs. Both are decent pain relievers. Acetaminophen is an analgesic and antipyretic, which means that it relieves pain and lowers fever. NSAIDs do a little more: they fight pain, lower fever, *and* reduce inflammation. If you have joint swelling and inflammation, your doctor will probably prescribe an NSAID. Today NSAIDs fall into two categories: older drugs such as aspirin and ibuprofen and the newer COX-2 drugs such as celecoxib (Celebrex®).

NSAIDs Problems

Acetaminophen and all other NSAIDs, including aspirin, ibuprofen, and the new COX-2 drugs, have two serious drawbacks. First, they are all irritating to the stomach lining. This means that even short-term use of any of these drugs can cause stomach irritation, gastritis, and ulcers. These drugs can so damage the lining of your stomach and small intestine that gastrointestinal bleeding and other serious complications can happen. Even slight bleeding is undesirable, because it can cause anemia and other problems. Serious bleeding from an ulcer is a medical emergency that can even cause death. Up to 30 percent of patients taking NSAIDs develop ongoing gastrointestinal symptoms.

Another big problem with all NSAIDs, with the exception of aspirin, is that they can raise your blood pressure.[2,3] This may not be a problem if your blood pressure is average or on the low side, but if your blood pressure is borderline high (140 over 90), the drugs could push you over the edge into high blood pressure. And if you already have high blood pressure, as do over half of all adults over age 65, the drugs could make it worse. That in turn could lead to greater risk of stroke, kidney disease, and heart disease.[4]

Acetaminophen Pros and Cons

If your pain is not accompanied by inflammation, your physician will probably suggest an initial trial of low-dose acetaminophen. That's because acetaminophen is less expensive than a prescription NSAID, and also because at doses below 2 grams (2,000 mg) per day it has fewer side effects. Of course, that doesn't mean that acetaminophen doesn't have some side effects of its own. Until recently acetaminophen was considered to be much safer than the NSAIDs. That's why trying it was almost always recommended first, even though it doesn't work very well in most people. Fewer than two in five acetaminophen users get sufficient pain relief (defined as at least a 20 percent reduction) from taking the *maximum* dose of 4 grams per day. Surprisingly, almost as many get *worsening* of their symptoms after taking acetaminophen! If you give 100 people suffering from OA pain some acetaminophen, about 35 will have a good response, 30 will not notice any benefit, and about 30 will actually feel worse.[5]

In 2000, the American College of Rheumatology, which establishes guidelines for the treatment of osteoarthritis, still listed acetaminophen as a first-line therapy for pain relief. I believe this recommendation will change soon in light of increasingly negative safety information and evidence that only a very small percentage of people can successfully use acetaminophen to control their OA pain in the long term.

Acetaminophen is a good pain reliever if it works for you and is safe for you. Unfortunately, trial and error is the only way to test whether you're one of the 35 percent of people who can benefit from its pain-relieving effects.

Even though acetaminophen was introduced into medical practice in 1873, and has been commercially available in the United States since 1955, researchers still don't know exactly how it works. For the minority of people who notice pain relief of at least 20 percent or more, acetaminophen is believed to work by blocking pain in the brain, not in the joints where the pain may be originating.

At the usual dosage of up to 2 grams per 24-hour period, acetaminophen is generally well-tolerated. But the more you take and the longer you take it, the more likely you are to have problems. You're especially vulnerable if you take a larger amount—up to the maximum daily dose of 4 grams per day—or if you take even a lower dose for many months or years.

Acetaminophen can cause liver damage and can harm the kidneys. In fact, heavy use of acetaminophen may be the culprit in as many as 5,000 cases of kidney failure each year in the United States.[6] Furthermore, a recent review of acetaminophen safety showed that daily doses at or above 2 grams (2,000 mg) can cause severe stomach bleeding.[7] This was a bit of a surprise, because acetaminophen was thought to be easier on the stomach than aspirin and other NSAIDs.

For decades, besides aspirin, acetaminophen was the only game in town. As a result, the medical community often turned a blind eye to its safety issues. Because acetaminophen has been around for so long, there were no major large-scale, long-term studies performed like the ones required to bring a new drug to market today. People needed pain relief, even if it was a bit risky.

Acetaminophen became available as a nonprescription, over-the-counter drug in the 1960s. Today it's found in nearly 200 over-the-counter products, including cold remedies and pain medications. It's also used in some prescription painkillers such as Percocet® and Darvocet®.

Debate over the safety of acetaminophen began in 1977. Beginning in 1988, the FDA convened expert panels as part of an ongoing review of over-the-counter (OTC) drugs, but the panels didn't get to acetaminophen until 2002. Even before that, however, many manufacturers had begun voluntarily adding a box on the label warning against liver damage caused by combining acetaminophen and alcohol, even though the evidence that this is really a risk is mixed and controversial.[8]

The FDA panel cited federal figures from 1993 to 1999 showing that acetaminophen overdoses resulted in 56,680 emergency room visits, 26,000 hospitalizations, and about 450 deaths per year. Most of these are related to suicide attempts, but unintentional overdoses alone accounted for 13,036 emergency room visits, 2,189 hospitalizations and 100 deaths each year. Add this to the cases of kidney and liver damage (even in low doses) and bleeding (in doses above 2 grams per day) and it's easy to see that the risks from acetaminophen should be taken very seriously. The FDA advisory panel recommended mandatory labels on acetaminophen products warning consumers of the possibility of liver damage from overuse.

Perhaps because of the frequent exposure to reassuring advertising, soft-voiced spokespeople, and smiling elderly television actors, most of the public does not understand the potential dangers of acetaminophen. The new warning labels will be a start.

A Closer Look at Acetaminophen

Why is acetaminophen so risky? Are the risks the same for everyone? In doses above 2,000 mg per day (one half of the maximum recommended dose), acetaminophen is a highly reactive chemical that can cause serious damage to the liver and kidneys.

Even if you're perfectly healthy and don't drink heavily, taking acetaminophen can still damage your kidneys and liver, especially if you take large doses regularly—as many people with arthritis do. A study in 2002 showed that accidental acetaminophen overdose is the most common cause of acute liver failure in America.[9] And some people are just more sensitive to the effects of acetaminophen and develop liver problems even from smaller doses.[10]

Even if you're not a drinker, and even if you don't have any symptoms, you might still have liver disease. One of the most common forms of liver disease, viral hepatitis, is present and without symptoms in several million Americans. Taking acetaminophen while you have undetected liver disease could make the problem much worse.

People who use acetaminophen on a daily basis over a long period are also at increased risk of kidney disease.[11] In fact, taking acetaminophen daily for a long time more than doubles your risk of kidney failure compared to people who don't take the drug regularly.[12]

The American College of Rheumatology and other medical organizations still recommend acetaminophen as the first-line treatment for minor pain of osteoarthritis. Because of the new safety concerns, this recommendation has come under fire recently.

Much of the information in the past related to the use of acetaminophen for osteoarthritis pain was based on short-term medical studies whose design did not meet current, more rigorous standards. In almost every instance, when a study using acetaminophen was funded by a company that had a vested interest in sales, the results somehow showed that when compared to an anti-inflammatory drug, acetaminophen was "as good" or "nearly as good" for treating pain. Not surprisingly, the opposite was also true. When a company that had a vested interest in sales of an anti-inflammatory drug funded a comparison, the NSAID performed better than acetaminophen. This is called publication bias—results that appear to be in favor of the company that funded the study.

One of the most well-designed studies ever performed on acetaminophen compared this drug to an anti-inflammatory drug on patients with documented osteoarthritis.[13] The findings—that acetaminophen didn't work as well—were no surprise to many physicians.

Most physicians are well aware that acetaminophen is rarely sufficient to control arthritis pain long term, that some patients actually have a worsening of symptoms using acetaminophen, and that acetaminophen has little, if any effect on inflammation (which causes much of the pain in osteoarthritis sufferers).

Acetaminophen, because of its easy availability and usefulness in some patients, still plays an important role in treating osteoarthritis. If it works for you, it's probably safer than the NSAIDs, unless you're a heavy drinker or have liver disease such as hepatitis or have kidney disease. But if your joints become more painful, swollen, and stiff even though you're taking acetaminophen, your doctor will probably look to the NSAIDs for their anti-inflammatory effect.

Making the Acetaminophen Decision

Should you try acetaminophen? Consider all these points first:

- If acetaminophen helps relieve your pain at a low dose, and you only need take it once in a while, it may be a good choice for you.
- Beware of taking more than one product containing acetaminophen: accidental overdoses can occur—and they may be fatal.
- Don't take acetaminophen if you have liver disease or consume on average three or more servings of alcohol per day.
- The more acetaminophen you take, the greater your risk of kidney damage, liver damage and fatal bleeding.
- Only one in three people get pain reduction of 20 percent or more using the maximum dose of 4,000 mg per day.

- About one person in four will feel worse taking acetaminophen compared to taking nothing.
- At doses above 2,000 mg a day, acetaminophen may be as likely to cause stomach upset and damage as low doses of NSAIDs.
- Acetaminophen is not a good choice in people who have joint inflammation.

If you do decide to take acetaminophen, there appears to be no reason at all to spend more on brand names. Less expensive generic acetaminophen is required by law to be exactly as good.

The Acetaminophen Bottom Line

It is unlikely the mainstream medical community will continue to recommend acetaminophen as first-line treatment for OA for much longer. It doesn't help many patients and there are serious safety concerns about long-term use. More importantly, acetaminophen only relieves pain—it does not help the health of your joints.

The NSAID Story

NSAIDs (nonsteroidal anti-inflammatory drugs) have become the most popular choice for physicians treating the pain of osteoarthritis. Developed as alternatives to the corticosteroids (which are *steroidal* anti-inflammatory drugs), NSAIDs were heralded as being slightly safer, albeit less powerful, than the naturally occurring cortico-steroids.

WHAT'S A STEROID?

Steroids *refer to a chemical structure that includes a specific group of attached, ring-shaped molecules. Steroids in the body generally refer to male or female hormones, which have effects on* *the sexual organs and bone and muscle building, or the family of corticosteroids, made by the adrenal glands that sit on top of the kidneys. Corticosteroids, such as Cortisol, are important in regulating our body's stress and immune systems. Synthetic corticosteroids such as cortisone and prednisone are powerful anti-inflammatory drugs and are sometimes necessary for very short-term use, or single joint injections only. Corticosteroids are great at reducing pain and inflammation, but they have some nasty side effects that make them downright dangerous—like depressing the immune system, thinning bones, increasing the risk of bone fracture, and impairing wound healing. When taken in high doses or for long periods of time (months or more), corticosteroids can cause hypertension, cataracts, diabetes, thinning and bruising of the skin, osteoporosis, and even mental disturbances. That's why a substitute for the corticosteroids, such as the NSAIDS, was so necessary—and so welcome.*

Aspirin is the most popular and best known of the NSAIDs. In fact, aspirin was being used long before the concept of NSAIDs was ever dreamed of. In 1758, the Reverend Edward Stone found that an extract from willow tree bark helped reduce fever and pain in 50 of his patients. The extract was studied and refined for years, finally emerging as a nonsteroidal anti-inflammatory that became known as common aspirin. Other NSAIDs were developed in the 1960s. First came indomethacin and then came ibuprofen.

Today, there are more than 100 different NSAIDs either on the market or being investigated. Over-the-counter (nonprescription) NSAIDs include aspirin, ibuprofen (Advil®, Motrin®, Nuprin®, and generics), naproxen (Aleve®), and ketoprofen (Orudis®). Prescription NSAIDs include a number of high-dose ibuprofen formulations. Drugs that are closely related to ibuprofen are also prescribed, including fenoprofen (Nalfon®), flurbiprofen (Ansaid®), ketoprofen (Orudis®), meclofenamate (Meclomen®), mefenamic acid (Ponstel®), and oxaprozin (Daypro®). Other prescription NSAIDs include diclofenac (Voltaren®), fenoprofen sulinac (Clinoril®), indomethacin (Indocin®), meloxicam (Mobic®), naproxen (Naprosyn®), and piroxicam (Feldene®). Which drug your doctor prescribes will depend a lot on the type of arthritis you have, which kind you have responded to in the past, how well you can remember to take medicine, and the best way for you to take it.

The latest generation of NSAIDs are the COX-2 inhibitors such as celecoxib (Celebrex®) and rofecoxib (Vioxx®). These new drugs have been hailed as a big step forward in painkillers, with fewer side effects than the older NSAIDs. As I'll explain later in this chapter, however, the claims haven't held up very well since these drugs were introduced in 1999. In many ways, they are no better or worse than older (and less expensive) NSAIDs.

LOW-DOSE ASPIRIN AND PAINKILLERS

Because aspirin helps make your blood a little "thinner" and less likely to clot, many older adults now take a daily low-dose (82 mg) aspirin tablet. Among the NSAIDs, only aspirin has the heart-protecting anticlotting effect. But what if you also want to take an NSAID to help with arthritis pain? What happens when aspirin is combined with these other drugs? In the case of acetaminophen and COX-2 drugs, the anticlotting effect of the aspirin doesn't appear to be affected—as long as the drugs are taken at least two hours apart. Ibuprofen, however, seems to block the anticlotting effect of the aspirin even when it's taken separately.[14] There's no evidence that glucosamine/chondroitin or ASU have any effect on low-dose aspirin therapy. If you need low-dose aspirin therapy and you also want to use painkillers—even over-the-counter ones—for arthritis pain, discuss the options with your doctor first. You may be at increased risk of stomach upset and gastrointestinal bleeding if you combine the drugs.

How NSAIDs Work

NSAIDs work by blocking the production of prostaglandins, hormone-like substances in the body that "cause" the pain and inflammation responses. Prostaglandins have many other important and necessary functions, however. They play a role in the regulation of blood pressure, blood coagulation, kidney regulation, and the secretion of gastric acid as well as the protective barrier in the lining of the stomach. Anything that interferes with the "bad" actions of the prostaglandins will hamper these "good" ones as well. That's why taking NSAIDs can interfere with vital bodily activities, triggering side effects such as:

- high blood pressure
- ulcers or stomach bleeding
- nausea
- cramps
- indigestion
- diarrhea
- constipation
- sensitivity to sunlight
- nervousness
- confusion
- drowsiness
- headache
- premature delivery in pregnancy
- asthma attacks
- swelling of the fingers, hands, and feet along with weight gain or urinary problems (these may all be signs of heart or kidney disorders and should be immediately reported to your doctor)
- anaphylaxis (a rare, severe allergic reaction characterized by difficulty in breathing or swallowing, a swollen tongue, dizziness, fainting, hives, puffy eyelids, fast and irregular heartbeat or pulse, or a change in face color. This is an emergency situation; you should immediately seek help if you experience any of these signs.)

The longer you take NSAIDs and the higher the dose, the more likely you are to experience these side effects. Sometimes, however, even one or two doses can trigger symptoms.

There is growing evidence that NSAIDs may inhibit the synthesis of proteoglycans, those important molecules that attract water to the cartilage.[15] In other words, the pills we take to block osteoarthritis pain may actually *decrease* the production of proteoglycans and make the arthritis worse.

On the other hand, when used for short-term relief from pain and inflammation, NSAIDs can be quite helpful. But by quelling pain these drugs can disguise or "mask" your osteoarthritis symptoms. You may believe that your condition is under control because your shoulder feels okay or your knee isn't as swollen. But the disease process *does* continue, whether you feel its effects or not. To make matters worse, some studies suggest that NSAIDs not only don't delay the progression of osteoarthritis, they may actually *hasten* it.[16,17]

I have a personal interest in the side effects of NSAIDS. My 98-year-old grandmother had been on various NSAIDs for years due to severe osteoarthritis of her knees. Unfortunately, she developed kidney problems from these drugs—I wish I had known about glucosamine/chondroitin and ASU sooner. They appear to work without measurable side effects, even with long-term use.

Should You Use NSAIDs?

To be fair, NSAIDs provide faster pain relief than either glucosamine/chondroitin or ASU, but the relief quickly plateaus and often diminishes with time. If your symptoms are severe, you may want to use one of these painkillers for a week or more in conjunction with glucosamine/chondroitin and ASU, and then taper off of the medication as the nutritional supplements begin to rebuild the cartilage matrix. Of course, you should check with your physician before beginning or changing any medicinal regimen.

NSAIDs may be a good choice for you if you need some additional pain relief and you have signs of inflammation (swelling, redness, warmth of a joint not due to infection). NSAIDs should be used only when absolutely necessary. Even in over-the-counter version they can be very dangerous drugs. Every year in America NSAIDs lead to 16,500 deaths and over 103,000 hospitalizations.

About half of the deaths from NSAIDs are from sudden bleeding, usually from a stomach ulcer caused by the drug. Unfortunately, only one in five people who develop ulcers from NSAIDs have warning symptoms such as nausea and pain before a serious bleed. Most people just start to bleed and pass out or die without warning.

Most other deaths from NSAIDs are from kidney and liver damage, high blood pressure, interactions with other medicines, asthma and allergy attacks, and several other causes such as destruction of bone marrow cells. If you already have kidney disease, liver disease, high blood pressure, or if you are allergic to sulfa drugs, use NSAIDs only if your doctor prescribes them and be aware of your increased risk of side effects.

Whether or not NSAIDs help with your pain is determined by trial and error. In general, about one in three people will notice a benefit from a particular class of NSAID. If you don't notice any benefit, your doctor will likely keep switching products until you find one that gives you pain relief. When it comes to NSAIDs, generic versions are exactly as good as name brand prescriptions. Don't waste your money on advertised brands.

Minimizing the Side Effects

Although side effects are common when taking NSAIDS, these unwelcome visitors can often be turned away by following these guidelines:[18]

- To reduce the risk of stomach upset (but not bleeding), take NSAIDs with food. It's often helpful to eat, take the pill, then eat again.
- To help prevent the development of ulcers while you're taking NSAIDs, your doctor may prescribe misoprostol (Cytotec®). If you're pregnant, your doctor will suggest a different medication.
- Drink at least eight ounces of water when taking tablets or capsules to keep the lining of the esophagus and stomach from becoming irritated.

- Don't lie down for 30 or so minutes after taking your medicine. Gravity helps assure that the pill passes through the esophagus to your stomach.
- Always take the exact dose prescribed by your doctor. Never double it, even if you miss a scheduled dose.
- Pregnant or breast-feeding women should not take NSAIDs (even one dose) unless specifically directed to and monitored by a doctor.
- Do not use alcohol while taking NSAIDS. Doing so increases the risk of stomach problems.
- Don't combine acetaminophen (such as Tylenol®) or aspirin with other NSAIDs unless specifically directed to do so by your doctor.
- Inform your doctor of all other medications you are taking, whether prescription or over-the-counter, so he or she can determine whether one drug will interact with another.
- If you are having surgery, inform your doctor or dentist that you are on NSAID therapy, even if it's just a low dose.
- Avoid driving or operating machinery when you are taking NSAIDS. The drugs may cause drowsiness, confusion, or dizziness in a small number of patients.
- Avoid direct sunlight or use a sun screen with a high SPF number. Your skin's sensitivity to sun may be increased during NSAID therapy.
- Using over-the-counter or prescription antacids or acid-blocker medications can mask the warning symptoms of serious stomach bleeding. Do not take these medicines in order to better tolerate an NSAID.

The COX-2 Inhibitor NSAIDs

You'd have to be living in a cave not to be bombarded with ads for the COX-2 inhibitor NSAIDs celecoxib (Celebrex®), rofecoxib (Vioxx®), and valdecoxib (Bextra®). Newer versions such as lumiracoxib, parecoxib, and etoricoxib have recently become available or will be soon.

Numbers one and two in pharmaceutical advertising in 2001, and among the top fifteen drugs in annual prescriptions, Vioxx and Celebrex were touted as the new and improved anti-inflammatories less likely to cause serious side effects. No claims were ever made that these drugs were any more effective at pain relief than traditional NSAIDs, and the research evidence has borne this out. Unfortunately, the COX-2 drugs have not lived up to their safety billing. In fact, serious safety concerns have arisen. In addition, there's some good evidence that using these drugs can cause you to lose more cartilage in your joints than you might by taking nothing at all, even if the drugs help relieve some pain.

The Operation Was a Success, But the Patient Died

Doctors and patients alike hoped that the highly selective COX-2 inhibitors would be a major breakthrough for treating arthritis pain. Sadly, the real-world testing of these drugs has been mostly disappointing. At best, they are only equal to generic NSAIDs in relieving pain. Among patients at the highest risk for developing intestinal bleeding and ulcers, these drugs are only slightly safer than generic NSAIDs. I became suspicious when my aunt suffered a life-threatening bleed after starting Celebrex and one of the surgeons who operated on my knee years ago had a stroke while taking Vioxx. I noticed in my practice, then confirmed by looking at the research, that only about one in three users of these COX-2 inhibitors actually get sufficient pain relief. The dropout rate for using these drugs, from treatment failure or adverse reactions, can be as high as 50 percent in the long term.

Recently the research has started rolling in and research scandals have appeared. All of the major studies of COX-2 inhibitors were funded by the drug companies and controlled by their employees and consultants. Some of the data reported to the FDA were not the same as what was published. Also, in almost every case, there was significant publication bias. The companies funding the research always managed to show that their product was somehow better than the competition. A good example is the study that supposedly showed Celebrex is safer than other widely used pain relievers because it causes fewer ulcers. This study, which appeared in 2000 in the prestigious and widely read *Journal of the American Medical Association,* showed that over a six-month period, patients who used celecoxib (Celebrex) did indeed have fewer ulcers and other gastrointestinal complications than patients who used high-dose ibuprofen or diclofenac (Voltaren®).[19] The problem is that the study went on for a year—and in the second six months, the celecoxib users had almost as many ulcer problems as the NSAID users.[20] A better designed study of rofecoxib (Vioxx), however, showed that this drug does reduce gastrointestinal complications compared to naproxen, but that the amount of pain relief was the same from both drugs.[21] A study in 2000 showed that rofecoxib provided about the same amount of pain relief from hip and knee arthritis as high-dose ibuprofen.[22] Another study in 2002 found that rofecoxib and celecoxib were somewhat better than high-dose (4,000 mg) acetaminophen at relieving the pain of knee arthritis.[23]

The bottom line? COX-2 inhibitors relieve pain about as well as but not any better than nonselective NSAIDs. Over the long run the COX-2 inhibitor celecoxib doesn't really protect you against gastrointestinal complications—you're almost as likely to have them as with the nonselective NSAIDs such as ibuprofen and naproxen. Rofecoxib may protect you against gastrointestinal side effects a bit better. Is the same amount of pain relief and a slight reduction of the risk of an ulcer enough to make the much higher price of the COX-2 drugs cost-effective? If you're at risk for ulcers or gastrointestinal bleeding (if you've have an ulcer before, for example), they might be worthwhile. To make the final decision, though, discuss the choice with your doctor—but not before you've read the next sections on some other very serious drawbacks to COX-2 drugs.

COX-2 Drugs and Heart Attacks

Just as disconcerting as the ulcer evidence turned out to be is new evidence revealing that the COX-2 drugs can cause coronary heart disease, including heart attacks. The major study that led to FDA approval

study for Vioxx showed a 400 percent higher heart attack rate compared to those in the study taking naproxen, a nonselective NSAID.[24]
The significance of this has been debated for several years. In 2001, a
study in the *Journal of the American Medical Association* showed that
people who took COX-2 inhibitors had a significantly higher risk of
having a heart attack or developing other forms of heart disease such
as angina compared to people who took naproxen.[25] This study was
confirmed by another in the well-known British medical journal *Lancet*
in October 2002. In this study, those taking rofecoxib (Vioxx) at the
highest dose recommended (50 mg) for more than five days were 70
percent more likely to develop coronary heart disease. This was no
small study—data was analyzed using records from 375,000 patients.[26]

Work with your doctor to compare the risks and expense of these
drugs to the pain relief you are likely to get. I think you'll decide
against them—and in favor of glucosamine/chondroitin and ASU.

As problems with the COX-2 selective drugs surfaced, the FDA
stepped in and forced the makers of the COX-2 inhibitors to change
their labeling, their advertising, and in some cases, their warning
labels. At least one COX-2 inhibitor drug launch was delayed, and I
would not be surprised if one or more of these drugs is taken off the
market in the future.

What disturbs me as much as the safety data is the growing evidence that the COX-2 selective drugs may impair the natural healing
response in cartilage. This is very serious, because it makes osteoarthritis progress faster, despite any potential pain relief. If this is
indeed the case, then we would have the rare and very unusual situation where an FDA-approved drug for treating a disease—in this case,
osteoarthritis—would worsen the disease process. Prescribing these
drugs would then be a clear violation of a doctor's oath to do no harm.
Imagine if we had a birth control pill that caused greater fertility, or a
cholesterol medicine that led to more heart attacks and strokes?

Alternatives to NSAIDs

If after reading all this you would very sensibly prefer not to take NSAIDs, there are some additional supplements (aside from glucosamine/chondroitin and ASU) that can help reduce inflammation naturally and safely. Many of my patients find that two oils, gamma linoleic acid (GLA) and eicosapentaenoic acid (EPA), and the dietary supplement Nexrutine® are often very effective.

GLA is an oil found in borage seeds, black currant seeds, and evening primrose seeds. The usual daily dose for treating inflammation is 1.4 grams a day. EPA is found in fish oil (and in fish) and in flaxseed oil. The usual daily dose for treating inflammation is 2.6 grams a day. Flaxseed oil has less EPA than fish oil, so you'll need to take more of it to get the equivalent amount.

Nexrutine is an herbal product made from the Amur cork tree (*Phellodendron amurensi*). It has been used as an anti-inflammatory in traditional Chinese medicine for centuries. Its action is in some ways similar to the COX-2 inhibitors, but with perhaps less risk of intestinal bleeding. In fact, there's some evidence that Nexrutine actually helps prevent ulcers. A number of trials are now under way; I look forward to the results. The usual dose for Nexrutine is 250 mg two or three times a day. Some people find that they need to double the dose to get relief.

Be sure to discuss using these supplements with your doctor before you try them.

Before Taking Any Medicines

Drugs are powerful weapons against distress. But they're not "smart bombs" that know exactly what to target. Many, many people have been harmed by medicines that destroyed the wrong target in the body. Physicians are supposed to make sure that patients get exactly the right medicine at the right dose at the right time and for the right reason. Unfortunately, that's not always the case. Sometimes doctors are unaware of a medicine's side effects or forget to ask which drugs you are already taking before prescribing a new one. The situation is getting even worse with the move toward managed care, for now many doctors are pressured or required to prescribe a limited number of drugs, even if another one may be better suited to your needs.

That's why it's up to you to ask questions—plenty of them—before agreeing to take any medicine. Insist that your doctor answer all your questions fully. Don't accept "don't worry about it" or "you wouldn't understand" for an answer. Here are some of the questions you should ask:

- Why do I need this drug?
- What are the possible side effects, from the most common to the very rarest?
- Who is most likely to have these side effects?
- What early signs will warn me that side effects may be striking?
- Is there another medicine better suited to my needs?
- Is there a generic version of the drug that would work just as well for me but costs less?
- How many times a day should I take the medication? When? Should I take it with food or water, or on an empty stomach?
- Are there any foods or drinks I should avoid while taking this drug?
- Are there any activities I should restrict or avoid while taking this drug?
- How soon should the drug begin working?
- How will I know it's working?
- Assuming it works, how long should I continue taking it?
- If it doesn't work, how long before we try something else?
- Is there a nondrug treatment I might try?

After you've questioned your doctor, be sure to tell him or her if you are already taking any other drugs, nutritional supplements, or other substances. To be sure you've told the doctor about everything you take, bring along a complete list that gives the names and dosages. Also mention whether or not you've had adverse reactions, allergies, or sensitivity reactions to *any* medicines or other substances. Even the smallest reaction may be important, so don't hesitate to speak up.

Remember: Doctors are sometimes quick to prescribe drugs, but every single drug has side effects. You are not required to swallow everything your doctor gives you. Feel free to ask questions. And if you don't like the answers, insist on hearing about other treatment options. *When it comes to your health, you're the boss.* You have the right to have all your questions answered completely and to your satisfaction before you make a decision.

If your doctor prescribes medicines for your osteoarthritis, ask about glucosamine/chondroitin and ASU. If your physician is not aware of these three nutritional supplements, show him or her this book.

8

EXERCISE THAT *HELPS,* NOT HURTS

Why is exercise so important?

Can exercise help damaged joints? Or does it actually cause osteoarthritis?

Does exercise strengthen bones?

Can exercise really prevent joint deformities?

Which exercises are best?

Why is stretching necessary?

How does exercise reduce my fatigue level?

How do I get started?

A 75-year-old retired high school teacher, Bill had lived an active life, working with teenagers, gardening, camping, backpacking, and acting as the neighborhood "fix-it" man. Anytime people in the neighborhood had a problem with their sprinklers or their plumbing or their gas heaters, they called on "good ol' Bill," who graciously came over to lend a hand.

Once he turned 70, though, the osteoarthritis that had bothered his left knee for some time started to get pretty bad. Luckily he wasn't teaching anymore—all that standing would have been impossible. And camping and backpacking were pretty much a thing of the past. At first he took these changes in stride. But before long he had to give up gardening and couldn't even walk halfway down the block to help a neighbor. A friend suggested he try water aerobics at the YMCA. He did, and the results were surprising. He told me, "Exercising in the water is great because it supports your weight. Since I've been doing it, my knee is a lot less stiff, I don't limp as much and some days it barely hurts at all. I guess exercise is sort of like greasing up a rusty door hinge and then working the grease in by opening and closing the door a bunch of times."

Bill's explanation of why exercise helps ease osteoarthritis symptoms is actually not too far from the truth. It may sound strange, but one of the best medicines for osteoarthritis is exercise. The right kind of exercise can ease your symptoms, help you to lose weight, and help to take a load off your joints. It also improves immune functioning and enhances your overall health. Even aerobic exercise, which is often thought to be too strenuous, can be beneficial to people with osteoarthritis.[1]

For a long time, doctors believed that exercise aggravated or even caused osteoarthritis, and they advised against it. Perhaps that's one reason why very few osteoarthritis sufferers exercise on a regular basis. That's a shame, for they're missing out on a powerful and often fun treatment.

The Importance of Exercise

We have a natural tendency to slow down when we're injured or sick, to stop our normal activities in favor of rest. And that's often the wisest course. But in the case of osteoarthritis, too much sitting around can be devastating. We're designed to be up and around most of the day, walking, stooping, gathering, hunting, or working the fields. Our bodies have built-in mechanisms to conserve energy and prevent starvation. Atrophy—the wasting away of unused muscle and bone to lessen energy expenditure—is one of those mechanisms. That's what happens to osteoarthritis sufferers who cut back drastically on exercise. Their muscles lose strength, tone, and flexibility. The range of motion in their joints becomes limited and their bones get thin, while their cartilage both thins and softens. When you stop moving, osteoarthritis progresses more rapidly.

Exercise helps to keep joints healthy. Even though glucosamine/

chondroitin sulfates and ASU rebuild cartilage while reducing osteo-arthritis symptoms, it's very important to continue exercising. Sure, you might have to modify your activities according to the needs of your joints, but as you'll soon see, there are many exercise choices available for people who have problems in almost any joint. Movement in any of its many forms, whether it be walking, biking, lifting weights, yoga, swimming, and so on, is now widely accepted as an important part of the treatment for osteoarthritis. It fights the debilitating effects of this disease in three major ways:

Exercise encourages the flow of synovial fluid into and out of the cartilage. Synovial fluid lubricates and nourishes cartilage; its very presence is believed to slow the progression of osteoarthritis. The constant movement of liquid into and out of the spongy cartilage keeps the cartilage moist, healthy, and well nourished. But without the pressure created within the joint by movement and exercise, the liquid will not flow in and out. This impedes nutrients from getting to the cartilage cells and hinders the elimination of waste products produced in the cartilage. Exercise helps to prevent this from happening by keeping joints "wet" and well nourished. (This helps explain why an osteoarthritis sufferer will often have the most discomfort right after a period of inactivity—the joint has not been nourished for a while. The phenomenon is sometimes called "movie-goer's knee.")

Exercise strengthens the supporting structures (muscles, tendons, ligaments) and increases the range of motion, shock absorption, and flexibility of the joints. Strong, well-toned muscles, tendons, and ligaments can bear the brunt of the force that crashes into joints as we move, while helping the bones support the body. In fact, the majority of the load that the joints bear can be transferred to these supporting structures, allowing the articular cartilage to maintain its integrity.[2] Without the stress-dampening effects of the muscles in your thigh, for instance, the simple act of walking down a stair or two could tear all of the major ligaments in your knees. The manner in which your muscles contract, not just the strength of the muscles, helps determine how well you can absorb shock in your joints. We used to think that when people with knee OA lost muscle strength in the thighs, it was because they avoided exercise, and thus lost muscle tone. We now know that the loss of strength *precedes* knee OA in many people. In other words, in women without knee pain or any sign of OA, those with less muscle strength in the quadriceps (the muscles in the front of the thighs) are most likely to later develop OA.

Exercise also allows us to move better—it gives us better biomechanics. Think of biomechanics as how well or smoothly the muscles and joints function. Different from strength, biomechanics is more related to the *coordination* and *timing* of movement. Someone with good biomechanics makes movement and exercise look easy, almost effortless. A good example is a skilled ballerina. Through training and practice, she jumps, twirls, and lands in a fluid and smooth motion. The force of this jumping and landing would quickly lead to injury, and perhaps OA, if the ballerina didn't have good biomechanics that to allow her muscles to contract and her joints to move just at the precise moment.

Recently researchers identified at least one of the reasons why exercise actually helps to relieve pain in osteoarthritis sufferers.[3] Samples of the joint fluid of osteoarthritis patients was removed from the knee before and after 12 weeks of simple isometric (muscle contractions without joint movement) exercise. Examination of this fluid revealed that the post-exercise samples had more thick hyaluronic acid, a key component for both lubrication and shock absorption in the joint. In addition, fragments of free chondroitin that had floated into the joint fluid were reduced, indicating that they were probably maintained better in the cartilage matrix. It's no wonder then why some people have an aggravation of their joint pain if they *don't* perform their regular exercises. Even skipping a day or two can cause some people to experience a worsening of their symptoms. I have called this phenomenon "exercise-dependent osteoarthritis."

And that's not all. Exercise's many other benefits to mind and body are so numerous that, if we didn't have hundreds upon hundreds of studies to back up the claims, you would think that they were pretty farfetched. Here's what we know exercise can do for you:

- improve your physical capabilities
- prevent joint deformities

- contribute to better emotional health
- reduce stress
- enhance sleep
- promote relaxation
- improve body composition (that is, gain muscle, lose fat)
- increase your resistance to other diseases
- improve insulin sensitivity and decrease the risk of developing diabetes
- build up a reserve capacity in the event of disease
- improve sexual function, satisfaction, and body image
- improve balance
- help you preserve your independence

Lack of regular exercise contributes greatly to the development of high blood pressure, obesity, diabetes, and heart disease. In fact, a sedentary lifestyle is second only to smoking as the most common cause of disease and death in the United States. Even the simplest of exercises can be tremendously helpful. The importance of walking or water aquatics was demonstrated by a study done at the University of Missouri. Of the 120 subjects, 80 had osteoarthritis. The participants were randomly assigned to two groups: one with an exercise program consisting of either aerobic walking or aerobic pool aquatics; the other a control group consisting of nonaerobic range-of-motion exercises. Each group met three times a week for an hour for a total of 12 weeks. The results were impressive. By the end of the study, the aerobic group showed significant improvement in aerobic capacity, walk time, and physical activity level, results that were much better than those for the range-of-motion group. In comparison to results from two drug studies, the exercise study participants had results that were at least as good.[4] They had fewer arthritis symptoms, but without the expense and risks of drugs and with all the added benefits of improved fitness.

If simple exercises can reduce pain and improve your ability to move, imagine what a full exercise program can do for you!

Exercise Strengthens Bones

Bones are not like the pillars holding up bridges or the steel beams inside buildings. The pillars and beams are static—they don't change. Bones are dynamic, not static, constantly changing in response to the changing demands made upon them. The *osteoclasts* in our bones continually tear down old bone cells, while the *osteoblasts* build new ones. In that sense bones are quite a bit like muscles, growing thicker and stronger in response to a heavier work load. In fact, obese people tend to have very strong bones because they have to support so much weight. (Gaining weight to increase your bone strength is not advised, however.)

Years of study have proven that regular exercise increases bone density, thereby making bones stronger. But not any exercise will do. The two kinds of exercise that help bones grow stronger and thicker are *weight-bearing exercise* and *strength training.*[5]

Weight-bearing exercise is simply related to gravity. This means that your bones have to hold you up, supporting your body weight while working against the force of gravity. Walking is a weight-bearing exercise for the feet, legs, and hips. Gravity has less and less effect as you move up the spine. For example, your neck has only the weight of your head on it, but your lower back must support the weight of the head, arms, and trunk. And your feet support the weight of everything. Generally, weight-bearing exercises work the lower body more than the upper body. (Although that's not to say that they are useless for the upper body, because it is taking on some of the load.)

The second kind of exercise that helps build bones and keep them strong is *strength training.* Also called resistance training, strength training involves repeatedly lifting or moving a load (weight) to the point of muscle fatigue in a limited number of repetitions (less than 15). Lifting free weights (dumbbells or barbells) and using weight machines and resistance devices like elastic tubing are all examples of strength-training exercises. You don't have to lift hundreds of pounds to improve your strength. For many, 5- to 10-pound weights are all it takes to get started. It's the form, or how well you perform the motion, that's key.

If the repetitions (number of times you lift the load) are limited by muscle fatigue to about 15 or less, the exercise is strength training. If you do more than 15 repetitions, the exercise becomes *muscle-endurance* training. Muscle-endurance training has its benefits, but isn't nearly as efficient at improving strength, muscle, and bone mass. If you want to do strength training and you find that you can do more than 15 repetitions of an exercise without muscle fatigue, it's time to increase the amount of weight rather than increasing the number of reps.

All about Exercise and Fitness

One of the primary goals of exercise is to improve fitness. There are nine types of fitness, including:

- strength
- aerobic capacity
- flexibility
- agility/balance
- sport-specific fitness
- muscle endurance
- power
- speed
- quickness

Only the first five types are required for health and the prevention of osteoarthritis. The others are mainly helpful for sports performance. Let's take a look at the types of fitness in detail:

STRENGTH

Are your legs strong enough to get you out of a chair? Can you easily lift bags of groceries? Can you do a chin-up using just your arms? Can you squat on the floor and raise yourself on one leg without help from your hands? You need strength to accomplish these tasks.

Strength is important for shock absorption in the joints, good bone health (prevention of osteoporosis), ambulation (the ability to move), reserve capacity in illness, weight loss, and weight control (since more muscle means higher metabolism). It's also important for preventing injuries; for instance, if you're not strong enough to lift something, you may injure yourself while lifting it improperly.

Exercises that improve strength include weight lifting (free weight and machines), rock climbing, heavy manual labor, yoga and Pilates classes, and any activity that causes your muscles to fatigue after a small number of repetitions.

Aerobic Capacity

Do you get winded walking up a hill? Can you walk a block? A half mile? A mile? After you've walked a long distance, does your heart pound so hard that you feel as if you must stop?

In a very simple sense, your aerobic capacity is your ability to keep moving, even when you're tired. Exercises that increase your aerobic capacity (including your breathing capacity and muscle endurance) have many other benefits, such as improving joint shock absorption and bone health (prevention of osteoporosis), weight control, and preventing stroke and heart disease and increasing your energy level. Brisk walking, running, biking, swimming, stair climbing, cross-country skiing, rowing, certain forms of dancing, many sports, plus aerobics and step classes can improve your aerobic capacity and cardiovascular fitness. Any activity that gets your heart rate up and can keep it up for at least 15 to 20 minutes consecutively is considered aerobic.

Flexibility

Can you sit on the floor with your legs together, knees straight, and touch your toes? When you bend down to pick up something, does your back only seem to bend in the lower region? Can you reach any spot that itches on your back?

Good flexibility is vital. Areas of relative inflexibility cause excess stress and force to be exerted on other areas of the body. This can lead to altered biomechanics, overcompensation, and osteoarthritis. And inflexible tissues are more likely to become strained or sprained.

Exercises that can improve your flexibility include yoga, stretching (all kinds), Pilates, ballet and other forms of dancing, and most of the martial art forms.

AGILITY/BALANCE

Do you have difficulty with balance? Do you have to grab on to furniture to steady yourself occasionally? Can you balance yourself while standing on one foot? With your eyes closed?

Good balance and agility allow you to maintain your activities with confidence as you age, and can help to prevent falls. Balance also improves your body's biomechanics by maximizing your ability to distribute shock for more effective absorption.

Exercises that improve agility and balance include yoga, ballet and other forms of dancing, most of the martial art forms, and sports that involve quick changes of direction (such as racquet sports).

SPORT-SPECIFIC FITNESS

Do you have a good-looking golf swing? Is your tennis serve fast, hard, and smooth? How well can you ski? Are you smooth and graceful down the slopes or on the verge of falling at any moment?

Sport-specific exercises are very useful for preventing injuries and, by extension, the osteoarthritis that they may induce. If you don't play a particular sport, you needn't worry about sport-specific exercises. But if you do, make sure your body is toned and prepared to play properly. Exercises that improve sport-specific fitness include the sport's standard drill exercises and playing the actual sport itself. Cross-training activities may help, too, such as playing soccer to help with the accuracy of football place-kicking.

MUSCLE ENDURANCE

How many push-ups can you do? Do your leg muscles tire more quickly than your breathing when you're climbing stairs? Do you say things like "I can walk forever, but my legs really get tired when I ski moguls"?

These are examples of muscle endurance: how long you can use your muscles at a low level before they reach fatigue. Usually this is not a major priority for normal health for most people, with one major exception. The risk of injury is much greater in people who have fatigued muscles. Many people who suffer ski injuries, for instance, report that these injuries occur at the end of the day, sometimes on the very last run they had planned to take. Their muscles were fatigued and they couldn't react as quickly.

POWER, SPEED, AND QUICKNESS

Can you run and jump quickly over a fence? How far can you throw a baseball or hit a golf ball? How fast can you run 50 yards? Can you get to the ball quickly while playing tennis or racquetball?

Although power, speed, and quickness are not necessary for modern-day survival, or to prevent osteoarthritis, they are essential for good performance in many sporting activities. Exercises that improve power include power lifting (not just lifting weights but lifting them quickly), football drills, and ballistic activities like plyometric training. Exercises that improve speed and quickness (how fast you can get up to speed, or accelerate) include sprinting of all types (whether on foot, on skis, on a bike, on skates, etc.) and specific speed drills. If you play sports competitively, then training to improve your power, speed, and quickness not only improves your performance but also can help you from becoming injured.

The Fitness Types Are Linked

The fascinating thing about the nine different types of fitness—and the five we're concerned with here—is that generally they are all lost at the same rate as we age and slow our activity levels. Balance, agility, strength, aerobic capacity, and flexibility are all lost by lack of use. Luckily, most kinds of exercise work on more than one area of fitness. For instance, walking can improve aerobic fitness and muscle endurance, while also maintaining and improving balance and agility. Playing a game of tennis may encompass aerobic fitness, agility/balance, flexibility, speed, and power. Yoga can help with balance, strength, and flexibility.

Aerobics, Jogging, Lifting, or What?

Even if you already have osteoarthritis and are limited in your ability to move one or more joints, there are many exercises you can do. But before choosing the exercises you want to do, think about your goals. An exercise program for osteoarthritis should do four things: strengthen the supporting structures of the joint, increase the joint's range of motion, stimulate the cartilage, and improve your biomechanics.

Strengthening supporting structures.   There are many ways to strengthen the muscles that work with your joints. Anything that involves lifting strengthens a muscle, from rearranging your closet to weight training. Walking, jogging, bicycling, dancing, and anything else that involves moving the body from place to place is good for the leg muscles. Swimming is an excellent toner for many muscles in the shoulders, back, arms, and legs. If you like walking but would like to give your arms a little workout at the same time, try carrying small weights in your hands or wearing wrist weights. And don't forget to consider a very important supporting structure: your heart. A good aerobic workout, the kind that gets your heart beating harder and your breath coming faster, strengthens your heart and circulatory system, allowing you to increase your level of exercise and, therefore, your level of fitness. It also helps you keep your weight under control and can give you an emotional boost.

Increasing range of motion.   Just using a joint is a simple way to hold on to whatever range of motion you currently have. Even if you have acute joint pain, you can still do range-of-motion exercises in a pool. Stretching is the best way to *increase* your joint's range of motion.

Gentle stretching helps to loosen up the muscles while making the tendons and ligaments more flexible and resilient. This, in turn, means that your joints will move more easily and stiffness will be reduced. Stretching also improves overall joint function, lessens joint pain, and releases pent-up tension. A more relaxed outlook on life and a better night's sleep are two extras that often accompany stretching's better-known benefits. So stretch regularly!

Strengthening, aerobics, balance, and stretching exercises can be performed safely and effectively by most osteoarthritis sufferers. However, *common sense and moderation are always the rules when exercising.* Ask your doctor, exercise physiologist, or physical therapist to tailor an exercise program to your specific needs and limitations. If you have an acute flare-up, your doctor may suggest that you do your exercises in the pool in order to take the weight off your joints, or he or she may ask you to stop exercising altogether for a short period of time. Remember that it's always a good idea to check with your doctor before returning to your normal exercise plan after you've had any problem.

Choosing the Right Exercise

There are three other important factors to consider when you're deciding which form of exercise will be best for you.

First is the importance of exercise in helping to prevent bone loss (osteoporosis). Choose an exercise that has a good balance between loading the bones to help prevent osteoporosis and loading the bones too much, which could lead to or worsen cartilage loss (OA). Jogging, doing step class, or even walking on a hard surface may be good to load the bones in the lower body to help maintain good bone density, but these may all be too much for someone with the symptoms of OA or someone who has a joint alignment problem (knock-knees or bow-legged). For any joint involved, there's a whole spectrum of activities that ranges from low joint impact to high. For knee and hip OA, for instance, the low end starts with activities such as water jogging/swimming and biking and moves up to moderate-impact activities such as weight training, walking, low-impact aerobic classes and on to high-impact activities such as jogging and sports where you need to jump or twist.

Next, consider the effectiveness of the exercise in weight control. You might not guess that full-out sprinting is the best way to control weight in the least amount of time. The problem is that, first, most people would get injured quickly, and second, sprinting is so mentally intensive that few could keep it up. Therefore, sprinting is a poor choice for most people, especially those with joint problems.

The Institute of Medicine guidelines now call for Americans to spend an hour each day doing some type of moderate exercise. It's easy to incorporate exercise into your daily routine. You can park farther away from your destination than you normally do and walk, or take the stairs instead of the elevator. Even gardening and house-cleaning are exercise.

As you become more fit, you can increase the intensity or duration of your exercise. As you get fitter, the amount of calories you burn in a one-hour workout goes up, which makes the exercise more efficient.

Finally, choose an exercise that interests you so you can stick with it long term. People often argue that one form of exercise is slightly better than another, because it burns more calories per hour or because it works more of your body. Oftentimes, the big picture is lost in the argument. Yes, cross-country skiing is more efficient than walking for burning calories and improving your fitness. But if you don't particularly like cross-country skiing, don't have access to the equipment, or don't do it frequently (and you can only do it in the winter anyway), then this is not a good exercise for you. An exercise you don't do is not very efficient at all. Most types of aerobic exercise are effective if done regularly in the proper manner. It's important for you to choose something that you enjoy doing and can do on regular basis regardless of the weather. In my experience, aerobic exercises that allow you to remain relatively still are the ones that people tend to stick with overtime. I've noticed this particularly with older populations. That's why stationary bicycles, either upright or recumbent models, are a good first choice for indoor exercise. You can easily watch television or even read while using a stationary bicycle or a treadmill. This helps prevent boredom and encourages you to continue to use this for long-term aerobic exercise.

One of the best ways to assure that you will maintain interest in exercise is to rotate among different activities in order to keep your experience fresh. I recommend to everyone that they have both outdoor and indoor activities so that weather, scheduling, or transportation don't get in the way of your daily workout.

Exercise and You

Each person is an individual and has individual needs. This is especially the case for someone affected by osteoarthritis. Even people who are the same age, height, weight, and sex, and who have the same joint affected (the knee, for instance), may require radically different exercise programs designed to meet their individual needs.

In general, focus most on those areas in which you're most deficient. What are they? You probably don't know—most people don't understand or can't interpret their body's needs. That's why an expert consultation with an exercise physiologist, physical therapist, or physician who specializes in sports medicine or physical medicine and rehabilitation (sometimes called a physiatrist) is a great idea. The experts can help you learn exactly what you should be doing for your specific problem and save you a lot of time, energy, and money.

Sometimes a specialist needs to gather some more data before making specific recommendations. This often includes a fitness assessment and perhaps even a body composition measurement. Let's look at an example. Jerry is a 47-year-old man who's been struggling with his weight and has had problems with osteoarthritis in his left hip due to an automobile injury. He has been going to the gym to exercise about two to three hours per week but has never had any professional assessment or advice. He's just been working out on his own. Most of the time, he's been lifting weights. He has some favorite exercises and has developed a weight-lifting routine that focuses mainly on the upper body.

Jerry went for an assessment by an exercise physiologist. The assessment included various tests for strength, aerobic capacity, flexibility, balance and also a body composition test using the most precise technique, a DEXA scan (which is also used to measure bone density). Jerry thought he was very fit because he was so strong. He could lift more weight than most of the other people in the gym. Much to his surprise, it turns out that Jerry had some significant deficiencies and a major imbalance in his fitness. Specifically, while he was flexible in some areas, he was extremely inflexible in his legs and hips. Furthermore, his aerobic capacity was in the lowest 10 percent for men his age. The biggest surprise came from his body composition test and bone density. Jerry had a lot of muscle, well above average for someone his size and age. But Jerry also had a lot of fat. This fat was concentrated in his trunk, which is a dangerous risk factor for diseases such as cancer, heart disease, and diabetes. In addition, Jerry's bone density test revealed that he was significantly below average in his hipbone density, even though he did not have any classic risk factors for low bone density.

After Jerry went through this testing, the recommendations for his exercise program change dramatically to concentrate on the areas where he needed the most work. Since his muscle mass and strength was not an issue, the exercise physiologist recommended decreasing the amount of time spent doing weight lifting and adding more time in low-impact aerobic activity. Jerry chose to use the elliptical trainer machine at the gym. This device simulates the movement of running, but since you don't lift your feet, there is very little impact on the cartilage in the hips. The motion on the hips is beneficial to stimulate cartilage, however, and it's weight-bearing enough to help with low bone density. Jerry was given a 10-minute stretching program that focused on the areas where he was most tight. We added two simple weight-lifting exercises for his legs that were designed to help strengthen the muscles around his hip joints and improve his bone density.

When I saw Jerry for a follow-up appointment four months later, he was in much better shape, even though he wasn't spending any more time on his exercise than before he received his new recommendations. His hip was feeling a lot better, he had lost a few pounds, and perhaps most important, a repeat body composition test showed that he was able to significantly decrease the amount of fat in his trunk.

What are your specific needs for exercise? In order to understand this, let's go over some more basic information as to what makes up a good exercise program.

- The time and effort involved.
- "Hassle factors" such as going to a gym or pool versus doing the exercise at home.
- Compliance issues. Is the exercise enjoyable enough for me to stick with it in the long term?
- What are my immediate, midterm and long-range goals?
- If obesity is an issue, more time doing aerobic activity may be needed.
- Those with poor strength may need to spend more time on strength training.

Designing Your Exercise Program

Exercise sounds like a simple matter—put on your sneakers and start sweating. However, finding the right exercises that strengthen your bones and supporting structures can be a little more complicated. Given that you may have already damaged one or more of your joints, strained the supporting structures, and possibly produced muscle imbalances, it would be wise if you began by enlisting the help of your physician, who can determine your general level of fitness and strength. He or she should evaluate your muscle strength, range of motion, and dexterity, as well as your ability to do simple tasks such as walking up and down stairs. The doctor will probably recommend a physical therapist or exercise physiologist, who will devise an exercise program for you based on your doctor's specifications. The physical therapist or physiologist will then guide you through a set of exercises designed just for you. Personal trainers are good to use if you have no significant problems, but they rarely have formal training in designing programs for people with limitations. And "cookbook" type programs for those who have no specific limitations should be avoided by those with joint problems.

Your physical fitness program should be set up so that you're gradually doing more intense exercise for longer periods of time, without straining or forcing to the point of injury. The program should include components to improve at least the first four types of fitness (strength, aerobic capacity, flexibility, and agility/balance). While exercising, keep these tips in mind:

- There is a cardinal rule for those who have osteoarthritis: *Never exercise through joint pain!* "No pain, no gain" refers to working through muscle soreness, not joint pain.
- Listen to your body. Stop exercising if you feel dizzy or sick to your stomach, if you're short of breath, or if your chest feels pained or tight.
- Don't overdo; you may injure yourself. There is a difference between doing a little more in order to improve, and pushing it to the point of injury. Learn to distinguish between the two. If you experience discomfort more than an hour after exercising, you've probably overdone it.
- Keep breathing while you exercise. You may be tempted to hold your breath when you exert yourself, but don't. Your body needs *more* oxygen when you exercise, not less. Your blood pressure shoots up when you strain and hold your breath. (Normal blood pressure is 120/80. Olympic weight lifters have been known to drive their blood pressures all the way up to 480/320!) Holding your breath will also cause lactic acid to accumulate in your muscles, which will increase the amount of muscle soreness you'll feel the next day.
- When you begin your exercise program, you'll probably feel tired, sore, and possibly out of breath. Take it easy, but keep going as long as you can. Eventually your body will adapt. Pretty soon, you'll be surprised at the things that you can do.
- Always cool down after exercising. Don't stop cold after exerting yourself. Instead, stretch, walk, shake out your legs and arms. Stay on your feet, if possible, since sitting down too soon after exercise causes your blood to "pool."

Now let's get into some exercise specifics. Walking, bicycling, and water exercises are the three approaches to fitness many osteoarthritis sufferers find both helpful and enjoyable. (Weight lifting is also critical to treatment but requires a bit more training and has a steeper learning curve.) Let's look at what each has to offer:

WALKING

Walking is perhaps the simplest and easiest aerobic exercise. Like other aerobic activities, walking makes your heart beat faster and your breath come harder. This, in turn, strengthens your cardiovascular system, burns fat, and generally tones and conditions your body. But you've got to do more than stroll at a leisurely pace to get your heart beating faster. You don't have to jog or run, but you do have to keep up a brisk pace. Aerobic walking can be as good for the body as running or bicycling. In fact, you burn the same amount of calories by walking as you would running the same distance.

Walking is a low-impact exercise, easy on the joints because they're not jolted by the force of your feet hitting the pavement the way they would be if you were running. (The exception is those who walk at fast paces. At speeds above 5 miles per hour, the impact to the joints is similar, whether walking or jogging.) Walking is inexpensive and requires little equipment other than a comfortable pair of shoes. It's also enjoyable, something you can do with a friend or loved one. Remember to keep the pace up, though, in order to get those all-important aerobic benefits.

To make sure that you're walking fast enough, but not too fast, try the talk-sing test: If you are able to talk while you're walking, without gasping for breath, but haven't enough breath to sing, you're moving at about the right speed. Walking in the "talk-sing" range offers many important benefits, including:

- increased endurance
- an overall sense of well-being
- greater flexibility in the hips, lower limbs, and possibly the back
- improved cardiovascular fitness
- greater lung capacity
- strengthened muscles in the lower extremities and back

- decreased body fat
- stronger bones in the lower extremities and hips
- improved control of your balance
- and, in many cases, less osteoarthritis pain

But before you put your feet to the pavement, remember to:[6]

- Consult your doctor. Ask him or her how long and how vigorously you should walk.
- Wear comfortable shoes, socks to absorb perspiration, and loose, comfortable clothing.
- Spend a few minutes warming up before you begin walking. Simple stretches can also help by loosening muscles, ligaments, and tendons, allowing them to absorb shock better while you walk. You can do arm circles; stretch your calves and some thigh stretches, but don't bounce or overdo it!
- After you've exercised, spend a few minutes cooling down. Now's the time to stretch for flexibility (I explain some stretching exercises later in this chapter).
- Gradually increase your distance. In the beginning you may want to take a couple of short walks per day rather than one longer walk.
- Walk on flat, solid surfaces—park trails, malls, asphalt or jogging tracks are your best bets for avoiding falls and injuries—until you become a pro.
- For safety's sake, walk during the day, not at night.

Most people with osteoarthritis can walk with little discomfort. But if you have severe hip, knee, ankle, or foot problems, walking may not be the best exercise for you. In this case it's especially important to get expert exercise advice.

BICYCLING

Bicycling offers many of the benefits of walking. But since your feet and legs aren't supporting your weight while you pedal, there's less stress and strain on those joints. People with more severe forms of osteoarthritis of the hips, knees, and feet may prefer biking to walking.

Bicycling is a limited weight-bearing exercise, so it's not the best approach to building bone strength and density. Still, bicycling is a great conditioning exercise. It can build up the muscles of the thighs (especially the quadriceps or the front of the thighs) faster than walking. These muscles are the ones that help you get up out of a chair, and they're critical for shock absorption. Moreover, biking is one of the main exercises recommended for those who have knee problems. The rotational movement is particularly beneficial to the cartilage and in the hips and knees. For some reason, the frequency of rotation between 70 to 90 cycles per minute stimulates the cartilage cells to produce more cartilage matrix. It's no surprise that even those affected by the most severe cases of osteoarthritis are able to maintain their joints by biking.

Whether you're indoors on a stationary bicycle or outdoors in the fresh air, remember:[7]

- Warm up for at least five to ten minutes on the bike before tackling any hills (on outdoor bikes) or adding resistance (on stationary bikes).
- Adjust the seat height so that your knees are just slightly bent when the pedal is at its lowest point.
- Make sure you can pedal without too much trouble. Adding resistance should be encouraged as you can handle it. (If using a stationary bike, do not add so much resistance that your pedaling speed drops below 70 revolutions per minute.)
- Pace yourself, especially in the beginning. About 15 to 20 miles per hour should be your initial maximum speed.
- If you have knee problems you may not want to climb hills on real bicycles, or use resistance on stationary bikes. Get the okay from your doctor first.

I've found that electric assist bicycles can be useful for those who like to bike outdoors, but just aren't able to go very far or go up hills. (See www.drtheo.com for the latest news on electric bicycles.)

WATER EXERCISES

Water exercises are popular with doctors, physical therapists, and patients alike because of the lack of stress and strain on the joints. Sometimes it's the only way that a patient with osteoarthritis can exercise without pain. And three key types of exercise—stretching, strengthening, and aerobic—can easily be done in the water.

You don't have to be an expert swimmer to participate in water exercises, because many of them are done with the help of a flotation device or while standing in the shallow end of the pool. And the benefits of water exercises are numerous, including:[8]

- decreased pain
- support for the body while offering resistance to the muscles as they perform the exercise
- easier mobility, which has the added benefit of improved emotional well-being
- relaxed muscles
- reduced joint compression
- social interaction, if you're in a class
- improved confidence levels as movement is increased
- improved coordination and posture
- a lower heart rate is maintained, so a higher level of exercise may be tolerated
- exercise can sometimes be continued even during a flare-up

As with any other form of exercise, consult your doctor before you begin a pool program. Remember that even apparently healthy people should not be alone in the water in case of an emergency. And if you use a colostomy bag or catheter, or have any physical impairments that make it difficult to get in and out of a pool safely, you should look into walking, bicycling, or other exercises instead of swimming.

One of the easiest ways to exercise in the pool is just to buy one of the inexpensive "noodle" flotation devices that kids enjoy using. By placing this long, cylindrical flotation device on your stomach and slightly leaning forward, or straddling it, you can be supported enough to go into the deep end of the pool and jog without your feet ever touching the bottom—this is called water jogging. Depending upon how fast you jog, this can be quite a workout. In fact, elite athletes who are trying to maintain their aerobic fitness at times of injury often utilize water jogging as a training aid.

WEIGHT LIFTING

There are so many specialized weight machines and kinds of free-weight exercises available today, it's almost certain that you'll be able to find at least some that are appropriate for you, no matter what your condition. Some of the machines can be a bit complicated, however, so get some instruction in how to use them properly. Weight lifting should not hurt your joints. If it does, you may not be doing the exercise properly, the seat may not be at the right height, or it may just be the wrong exercise for your condition. Get help and advice from an expert, and always listen to your body!

When trying a new exercise, perform the motion with little or no weight until you can do it with the proper form. Then begin to add weight, but don't worry about how many pounds you are lifting. The point is to help overcome or prevent osteoarthritis by increasing your muscle strength, not to win an Olympic gold medal. If you can only lift one pound in the beginning, that's fine. Don't strain by trying to lift 100.

You may not want to push yourself to fatigue the first time you do the exercise, for you may be very sore the next day. The soreness is usually a problem for beginners and goes away after repeat sessions of doing the same exercise. As you become familiar with the exercise, increase the amount of weight so that you reach fatigue with about 15 repetitions. Add some more weight and repeat the exercise to fatigue. You will now have done two sets. The first set, with more repetitions, allows you to warm up a bit to prepare for the heavier set. Adjust the number of sets that you do to your muscle-fatigue level. Some days you may need two sets, other days three sets to get the same feeling of fatigue. As long as your joints are not in pain, two sets are better than one, and three are better than two.

When you first start, you may want to limit the number of different exercises you do to about six, making sure that you're working both the upper and lower body. Two sets of six exercises should take only about 20 minutes. As you progress, add new exercises into your routine, and rotate them. Once you know what you're doing, and have a number of weight-lifting exercises to perform, your time is better spent by doing one set of many exercises compared to two or three sets of only a few exercises. Weight lifting using proper technique is one of the most efficient ways to help your joints and improve your bone density.

Always remember to exhale during the phase of lifting that has you straining the most. For example, if you're doing the bench press, exhale as you push the weight away from your body, then inhale as you let the weight back down to your chest.

STRETCHING

Stretching is an indispensable part of any good exercise program, but it is especially important to those people with osteoarthritis. If you stretch correctly, you can reap huge benefits. But if you do it incorrectly, you can do an awful lot of damage. Always be careful when stretching, and keep the following guidelines in mind:[9]

- Never stretch a cold muscle; always warm up first. Do your stretching at the *end* of your exercise routine, after you've broken a sweat and have engaged in some aerobic exercise, unless you are playing a sport. Little or no gain in flexibility is made if you stretch first with cold muscles.
- Make sure that you are in the correct position when stretching. It's best to join a class or have an instructor present to make sure that you're not stretching a muscle in the wrong way. Improper stretching can do more damage than good. For most stretches you want to be down on the floor so you can relax your body, especially the area you are stretching. If you don't relax the area you're stretching, your muscles will tighten slightly and you won't make much progress.
- Once you are in the correct position, stretch as far as you can without straining or forcing, then hold your maximum position for 30 seconds. In time, you can increase the hold to 45 seconds.

- Never "bounce" in your stretch; don't keep popping in and out of your maximal stretch. For the best results, relax into the stretch and hold that position. Bouncing can tear muscles, tendons, and ligaments. It also tells the muscles to tighten up just when you want them to relax.
- Don't hold your breath while stretching. Your muscles need the oxygen. Keep breathing, slowly and deeply. Exhale as you try to stretch farther.
- You can triple the effectiveness of your stretching sessions by using PNF (proprioceptive neuromuscular facilitation). Here's how it works: Get into your stretch, as far as you can comfortably go, and hold it. Then contract the muscles in the area you are stretching, without moving the joint. Hold this contraction for 5 to 8 seconds. Then relax the muscle, exhale, and you'll find that you can stretch even farther!
- Stretch at least three times a week, for 20 minutes per session. Stretching two days a week will generally allow you to maintain your current flexibility. Three or more days should bring about improvement.
- Stop if you feel any pain. Pain means you're damaging tissues. You should feel the stretch, but not pain.
- Form is everything. Don't cheat your stretch by contorting your body or using other joints to compensate for inflexibility.
- If you feel any unusual pains or sick in any way, stop and see your physician.

If your joints are quite stiff and you're not used to stretching, you may want to begin by working with a physical therapist, or join a special exercise class for arthritis sufferers. But once you've built up some flexibility, joining a yoga class or the stretch class at your local fitness center may be just the thing to keep you motivated. Feel free to try different classes until you find one that is both challenging and fun and has an instructor you trust.

There are several good stretches that you can do to loosen up your muscles, tendons, and ligaments and increase your flexibility:

For your back and the back of the upper thighs: Sit on floor with legs apart, arms at your sides. Bend forward and grab your left knee with both hands. If you can bend further, slide your hands down your leg as far as possible. When you have reached your maximum stretch, hold for 30 seconds without bouncing. Slowly bring your upper body to an upright position. Then repeat with your right knee. Spread your legs farther apart and repeat the exercise.

For shoulders: Stand or sit erect. Lift your right arm straight up, then bend it down and behind your head until your right hand touches your upper back (at the opposite shoulder blade, if possible). Reach your left hand over your head, grab your right elbow, and gently pull your right elbow toward your left shoulder. You should feel a good stretch in your right shoulder and upper arm. Hold for 15 seconds. Release. Repeat with other arm.

For lower back and hips: Lie on your back on the floor. Bend your right knee and bring it up toward your chest. Place both hands behind your knee and gently pull it toward your chest. Hold at your maximum stretch for 15 seconds. Repeat with other knee.

For calves: Stand a foot or two away from a wall or sturdy piece of furniture. Keeping your body straight (don't bend at the waist), lean forward, and brace yourself against the wall or furniture. Keep both heels on the ground (very important!). Slowly press both hips forward until you feel the stretch in your calves. If you don't feel the stretch, stand farther away from the wall or furniture and try again.

Fronts of thighs: Lie facedown on a mat or carpeted surface. Bend your right knee, grabbing your foot with your left hand. Hold for 30 seconds. Repeat with the other leg.

These are just a few of the countless stretches you can do. Ask your doctor or physical therapist for more. My book *Maximizing the Arthritis Cure* includes a detailed stretching program, complete with pictures and written instructions.

SPECIALTY AND MIXED-FORM EXERCISES

Yoga, Pilates and t'ai chi are three of my favorite exercise methods for those suffering from or wanting to prevent osteoarthritis. These exercise disciplines are very efficient, because the movements encompass elements of strength, balance, and flexibility simultaneously. These forms of exercise are wonderful for improving your biomechanics—and they're fun to do.

Yoga

Today yoga is becoming an increasingly popular form of exercise, especially for people with joint problems. This ancient system, first developed in India some 5,000 years ago, yoga integrates mind, body, and spirit. There are a number of different schools of yoga based on traditional Indian practice. There are also now a number of hybrid forms that combine yoga with other forms of exercise or use yoga exercises as part of an aerobic workout.

The traditional postures (asanas) of yoga are great for stretching, strengthening, and toning your body. Because most postures are easy on the joints, people with OA can usually do most them. And because there are so many postures, you can easily find those that put the least stress on a joint that may be aching. By working with an experienced yoga instructor, you can also choose postures that will help improve your biomechanics. Yoga movements can be done standing, sitting, or lying. No matter what the movement, it is always done slowly and thoughtfully. Each yoga posture focuses on a particular part of your body. A good yoga program combines a series of postures that exercises the whole body.

There's no "official" school of yoga, and although there are many different styles the fundamentals are pretty much the same. You can learn the basic postures from any of the excellent books and videotapes on the subject, but I recommend working with an experienced instructor to find the postures that are best for you and to learn how to do them properly. Yoga is so popular today that it's easy to find a class that is right for you at your local health center or through a private studio. The best class for you is the one in which you feel most comfortable. A good instructor will challenge you to improve but not push you beyond your capabilities. As you progress, you can move up to more difficult postures.

PILATES

Another exercise system that has become very popular recently is the Pilates technique. These exercises were developed by a European fitness guru named Joseph Pilates during World War I as a way to help rehabilitate wounded soldiers. Over the years, the technique has been refined and expanded into exercises that can be done by anyone, regardless of age or fitness level. Pilates exercises combine aspects of yoga, dance, gymnastics, and breathing techniques. The exercises are done on a mat or by using specialized machines. Mat exercises are usually performed as part of a class, but can be done alone. Learning to use the machines almost always requires one-on-one sessions with a certified instructor, especially at first; later, you can move on to semi-private or small-group classes.

The beauty of Pilates is that the exercises can be geared to accommodate people with joint limitations, making it an outstanding form of exercise for osteoarthritis sufferers. The exercises are designed to improve strength, flexibility, and core stability (strong abdominal and back muscles). As you build up strength and improve your range of motion, you can make the exercises more challenging.

You can learn how to do the mat exercises at home from a Pilates videotape, but the machines aren't really meant for home use. If you're interested in Pilates, the best way to get started is with a certified instructor at a local fitness center or private studio. To find a certified instructor near you, check with the Pilates Method Alliance (www.pilatesmethodalliance.org, or call 866-573-4945).

T'AI CHI CHUAN

You've probably seen photographs from China showing dozens or hundreds of people doing t'ai chi chuan exercises in parks. This ancient system is very popular throughout Asia, and it's becoming increasingly popular in the western world as well as a low-impact form of exercise. T'ai chi, pronounced "tie-jee," means "supreme ultimate fist," but that literal translation gives a false impression. Although t'ai chi is considered a martial art form, it's a very peaceful one designed to create quiet strength and balance in movement. T'ai chi is based on the belief that good health comes from balance and a constant flow of energy (*chi* in Chinese) through the body. A t'ai chi workout is a series of movements and postures that flow easily and fluidly from one to the next. The movements are slow, circular, and continuous, so they gently exercise muscles all over your body. As you do the exercises, you move fluidly from one posture into the next and continually shift your body weight, contract and relax your muscles, turn from side to side, and change body angles. The gentle flow of the exercises means there's no strain on any part of your body or on your joints. Moving smoothly from one posture to the next is very helpful for building leg strength, improving the range of motion in your joints, and improving your overall awareness of your body.

T'ai chi chuan workouts can be as simple or challenging as you wish. If you get interested in this form of exercise, you can learn the "push hands" technique. This helps you learn to move in response to a partner. It's mentally and physically challenging and helps you develop a better sense of how to use your body weight, muscles, and center of balance.

Today many health centers and private studios offer t'ai chi classes. As with any exercise program, find a compatible instructor and learn the basics and proper form by taking classes. After that, you can do t'ai chi at home, but part of the fun of the program is doing it with a group.

Getting Started

"I love the *idea* of exercise," a veteran couch potato once said to me, quite seriously. "It's actually *doing* it that I can't stand."

That's a common complaint. We all understand why exercise is good but find it hard to get started. Well, the key is simply to *get started*. And to help you do this, let's sweep aside the common arguments against exercise.

- *I haven't exercised for so long, I won't be able to do it.* Don't worry about it. Your doctor and your physical therapist will develop a special exercise program that's geared to your capabilities.

- *Exercise hurts.* You may be a little sore or stiff in the beginning, as your body adapts to the new movements and demands. But exercise, properly done, should not be painful. Pain means that you're either overdoing it or doing it incorrectly. Tell your doctor or therapist about any discomfort or continuous pain.
- *It takes too long to see results.* Ask your doctor or physical therapist to design a program that allows you to meet small goals quickly and consistently. A little success can make you a convert.
- *There isn't enough time to exercise.* If you haven't time for a half hour of walking or bicycling, followed by a warm-down and stretching session, remember that several short exercise periods can be just as effective as one longer period. Take advantage of lulls during the day to squeeze in a little exercise. Ask your doctor or physical therapist for exercises you can do while you're at work, standing in the bank line, or sitting in your car in a traffic jam. Seize any brief moment to loosen your joints and get fit. Even simple things like standing on one foot while you're brushing your teeth can help you with balance.
- *Exercising is boring.* Some exercises *will* bore you. So will some foods, movies, and books. The trick is to find one or more types of exercise that you enjoy. If you love the outdoors, walking or bicycling are excellent choices. If you love the feeling of being in water, swimming or water exercises may be for you. If you prefer to be indoors, yoga or dancing may be just right. Try exercising with a friend or family member. Join an exercise class. Listen to your favorite music during exercise. Walk through a park instead of around your neighborhood. Whatever exercise you do, make it as pleasant and enjoyable as possible. There's an exercise just right for you. If you look, you'll find it.

Quick Tips to Improve Exercise Motivation

Let's face it—there will some days when you'll need a little extra motivation to get yourself moving.

- *Get a workout partner.* If someone is waiting for you on the corner at 5:30 A.M., you'll be more likely to get up and out instead of sleeping in and skipping your workout.
- *Keep an exercise log.* This can be as simple as placing a red X on a calendar on the days you exercise, or it may be as complex as jotting down the specifics about your workout in a notebook.
- *Get new clothes/shoes/toys.* Without busting your budget, treat yourself to those bicycle shorts or that aerobics leotard you've always admired. Devices such as a heart-rate monitor can also be very motivating
- *Train for a competition or an event.* If you've got a goal, you'll work harder.
- *Do cross training or seasonal training.* This helps prevent boredom and works different parts of the body in different ways. Always make sure you've got an indoor activity to do in case of bad weather.
- *Keep equipment in plain sight.* Don't hide your tennis racket in a distant closet. Keep it out, where you can see it as a reminder to get moving!
- *Work out in the morning.* If you work out first thing in the morning, you'll have gotten your exercise in, no matter how busy your day becomes. The energized feeling you'll get from the workout will last all day.
- *Combine your workout with work.* Many people walk or bike to work or find ways to do some exercise during their lunch hour.
- *Ease up on days when you're not feeling strong.* You don't always drive a car in fifth gear; sometimes you have to downshift. On your "down" days, doing just a few minutes of exercise is far better than skipping it completely.
- *Subscribe to a magazine.* For about $1.50 a month, you get a reminder to exercise and some new ideas for things to do.
- *Try the 5-Minute Rule.* On days when you just don't feel motivated, plan on exercising for just 5 minutes. If you still don't feel like exercising after 5 minutes, quit. Most of the time, though, you'll start feeling invigorated and you'll continue.

Get Started!

Some people are reluctant to exercise because they fear they'll "wear out" their joints or damage them further if they already have osteoarthritis. Their fears sound reasonable, but they're not supported by the facts. Most scientists and doctors believe that even vigorous exercise *does not* cause osteoarthritis to develop in normal joints. In fact, it's just the opposite. The flowing of synovial fluid into and out of the cartilage from exercise *counteracts* damage in normal joints. When it comes to your joints, it's truly "use it or lose it."

Exercises that involve high stress-repetitive movements, such as pitching a baseball hundreds of thousands of times, can trigger *secondary osteoarthritis*. Those who engage in sports at highly competitive levels with injured joints are also at an increased risk for developing osteoarthritis. The bottom line is this: Use your common sense when exercising. Avoid specific exercises or activities that place abnormal stress on your joints. But *do* find some kind of activity that feels comfortable and start moving! Although glucosamine/chondroitin sulfates and ASU will help rebuild damaged cartilage, you need to exercise regularly in order to ensure good joint health.

——9——
HEALTHY EATING REALLY COUNTS

*How does my body weight affect
my osteoarthritis?*

*How can I reduce my osteoarthritis symptoms by
changing my diet?*

What is the "antioxidant connection"?

What foods can cause or reduce inflammation?

*How can fish oils help ease
osteoarthritis symptoms?*

*What can borage seed or evening primrose oil do
for osteoarthritis?*

*What role do bioflavonoids play in an
osteoarthritis diet?*

How can food allergies affect my arthritis?

Do other "arthritis diets" help?

You've heard all the clichés: "You are what you eat." "Food is the best medicine." "Your body is like a car and it needs the best fuel in order to run properly." Like most clichés, these are based on fact. You body is made up of about 75 trillion cells. Every day, billions are destroyed and billions more are formed. We use what we eat to create these new cells while providing building blocks for the existing cells to function. What we choose to put into our bodies can either strengthen or weaken us, making us more or less healthy while increasing or decreasing the symptoms of disease. This chapter tells you how to fuel your body with health-enhancing foods, some of which can lessen and may even help prevent some of the symptoms of osteoarthritis. If you follow these dietary guidelines, you'll also be beefing up your immune system and lowering your chances of getting heart disease, cancer, stroke, and diabetes—some of America's biggest killer diseases. We'll also discuss the essentials of a good diet, foods that may help to prevent or slow osteoarthritis, and the use of antioxidants and other supplements. We'll start, however, with the key issue of weight control. Maintaining a healthy body weight is vital to *preventing* and treating osteoarthritis.

Weight Control and Osteoarthritis

More than 100 million Americans—65 percent of all adults—are now considered overweight (at least 10 to 30 pounds above their ideal weight). Of that number, more than 30 percent are obese (more than 30 pounds overweight). Childhood obesity has almost tripled in recent years, from 6 percent in 1980 to over 15 percent in 2002. And according to the Federal Trade Commission (FTC), Americans spend over $30 billion a year on weight-loss products.

Staying slim isn't a guarantee that you won't get osteoarthritis, but putting on weight is almost a guarantee that you will, especially if you're a woman. Dozens of scientific studies have looked at the relationship between weight and arthritis, and they're all in agreement. If you're overweight, your chances of arthritis of the knee or hip are much greater than those of someone of normal weight. If you're obese, your odds of arthritis are even greater.

The connection between being overweight or obese and having arthritis, especially arthritis of the knee and hip, has been shown in a number of excellent studies. The heavier you are, the greater your risk. One well-known study from the 1980s found that the heaviest men have about 1.5 times the risk of knee arthritis as the lightest; among women, the heaviest have over twice the risk of knee arthritis as the lightest.[1]

In a follow-up study in the 1990s, researchers determined that every 10 pounds of extra weight increases your risk of arthritis by 1.4 times.[2]

The obvious link is that increased load on the weight-bearing joints, especially the knees and hips, can cause the cartilage to break down. The damage isn't just to the weight-bearing joints, however. Obese people also develop OA more often in their non–weight-bearing joints, such as their fingers and hands, compared to their slim counterparts. Researchers think this is because some substance that causes joint cartilage destruction, as yet unidentified, circulates in the blood of obese people.

Unfortunately, this leads to a vicious cycle: The heavier you are, the more likely you are to have OA, which reduces your ability to exercise, which leads to more obesity. Add depression (see chapter 10) into this cycle and we really have ourselves a challenge. If this wasn't enough, being overweight is a serious risk factor for Type 2 (adult-onset) diabetes, and being obese put you at even greater risk. Being overweight or obese *and* sedentary makes the risk even greater. Why is this important? Because diabetes is a risk for osteoarthritis as well. People with diabetes often have diminished nerve function—including the nerves that lead to the joints. Over the long term, people with diabetes can develop *diabetic neuropathy*, a oftentimes painful disorder that results in diminished sensation. Without full sensation to the joints, diabetics with neuropathy are unable to make the small corrections in balance and joint movement necessary to prevent the joint cartilage from being overloaded, even from everyday activities, such as walking on slightly uneven terrain. The result is an accelerated breakdown of the joint.

Here again we have a vicious cycle. Overweight, diabetes, diabetic neuropathy, joint damage, osteoarthritis, less exercise, more obesity, worsened diabetes, and so on.

As the American population—and people around the world as well—continue to get fatter, the incidence of arthritis will only continue to rise. So will the incidence of deadly heart disease, cancer, and diabetes.

Weight Loss Helps Arthritis

Just as we know being overweight contributes to arthritis, we know that losing weight can help prevent it from developing and make it easier to treat if it has. If you're not overweight, so much the better for your arthritis (to say nothing of your overall health). If you're overweight, losing those extra pounds is an important part of the Arthritis Cure. You don't have to go on a crash diet and lose a lot of weight rapidly. That would probably harm your health more than it would help, anyway, and just about everyone who tries to lose weight this way ends up gaining it back and then some. I recommend just the opposite: The slower you lose weight, the better.

Slow weight loss indicates that your diet and lifestyle are improving and can be maintained for the long haul. The best weight-control program combines two things: A wide variety of nutritious foods in reasonable portions along with moderate daily exercise. Any diet that promotes quick weight-loss, especially if the program doesn't also incorporate exercise, should be a warning sign to you that it is not effective in the long run, will keep you constantly obsessing about food, your appearance, and your weight, and is most likely unsafe for your long-term health. Besides, it will likely waste your money.

Lose Weight the Delicious Way

Too often, dietary advice is negative: Eat less, don't eat certain foods, stay away from junk food. A positive approach is more helpful. The easiest way to lose weight is to incorporate into your daily diet healthy foods with a good ratio of nutrients to calories.

That's easy to say, but what about some practical guidance? Fortunately, we have plenty of evidence for the benefits of a specific way of eating that provides a diet rich in high-quality nutrition, variety, and rich taste. It's called the Mediterranean diet.

The traditional diet that people have eaten in Mediterranean countries such as southern Italy, Greece, Crete, and southern France is considerably different from the standard Western diet. The main features of this diet include the following:

- Dietary fat is relatively high and comes mostly from olive oil. In the Mediterranean diet, 35 to 45 percent of calories come from fat, as opposed to the recommendation of 30 percent or less in the standard Western diet. But there's less saturated fat and trans fat in the Mediterranean diet.

- Protein comes from lots of fish, some poultry and pork, moderate amounts of cheese, and a little red meat.
- Carbohydrates come from fresh vegetables, beans, legumes, nuts, whole grains, and fresh fruit. Pasta, rice, and potatoes are eaten in small portions; whole-grain breads are preferred.
- Wine in moderation. A glass or two of wine each day has been shown to have some valuable health benefits—but only for people who aren't adversely affected by alcohol. You might have a medical condition, such as liver disease, that means you should avoid alcohol, or need to take medications that don't mix well with alcohol, or you might not be able to control your intake.
- Processed foods, snack foods, and convenience foods are eaten rarely if at all.
- Physical activity plays an important part in the Mediterranean diet.

There's been a lot of interest in the traditional Mediterranean diet recently because some excellent research shows that it offers major health advantages. In addition to helping you achieve and maintain a healthy weight, the Mediterranean diet helps prevent cancer and heart disease. In countries where the traditional diet is still followed, rates of breast cancer, for instance, are considerably lower than they are in United States.[3]

Unusually for nutrition science, the evidence we have for the value of the Mediterranean diet comes not only from epidemiological studies (studies of large groups of people) but also from carefully controlled prospective clinical trials that compare smaller groups to a control group. The classic study showing the value of the diet comes from the Lyon Diet Heart Study, which compared the fates of a large group of people who had had heart attacks. The group was randomly divided. One group was told to eat the traditional higher-fat Mediterranean diet; the other was told to eat the standard low-fat "heart-healthy" diet. Over the five-year study period, the group eating the

Mediterranean diet had fewer second heart attacks, was healthier overall, and had fewer deaths than the low-fat group.[4] (The Mediterranean diet has also shown benefits for rheumatoid arthritis—I'll discuss this more in chapter 12.)

Why the Mediterranean Diet Works

The Mediterranean diet works not simply because olive oil is the main source of fat. The diet also helps because of the fairly large amount of fish and the wide variety of fruits and vegetables, along with beans, legumes, nuts, and whole grains. In addition, you'll notice that the diet is low in simple sugars and sweets and processed foods. This eliminates just about all the dangerous trans fats. And because the diet uses very little red meat, eating the Mediterranean way means you consume only small quantities of foods that will result in arachidonic acid production, the precursor for inflammation (I'll explain more about this crucial subject later in this chapter).

Losing Weight and Keeping It Off

Following stringent diets, especially those that are very low in calories or fat or are based upon just a few foods, doesn't work for long-term weight loss. You may lose weight initially, but once the "diet" is ended, the pounds pile on in a hurry, and you may end up with more body fat than before you started. People who fall into the "yo-yo" trap of dieting, losing weight then gaining it back over and over again, become fatter and have a higher mortality rate than those who remain at a constant weight, even if that weight is high. In the long run, it's what you do on a daily basis that makes the difference. That's why it's important to adopt a sensible, flexible, and easy-to-follow eating plan.

How do you get control of your weight? Most people who have successfully lost weight and kept it off have certain characteristics in common. They include:

- *Making changes for themselves, not to please others.* Internal motivation is the key. *You* have to want to lose weight, keep fit, and reduce your osteoarthritis symptoms. You can't do it just because your spouse or your best friend has nagged you into it.

- *Focusing on fitness.* Rather than looking at numbers on a scale to see how well you're doing, focus on how much farther you can walk each day, or how many more repetitions of an exercise you can do than you did when you started. A formerly obese person who can now run a seven-minute mile rarely continues to have an obesity problem.

- *Doing at least some exercise each day.* Keeping your body in motion raises your basic metabolic rate and burns calories faster than before, even when resting! The more you exercise, the more calories you can take in while still losing weight. And because muscle is more metabolically active than fat, the more muscle you have, the higher your basic metabolic rate is and the more calories you burn.

- *Never skipping meals.* Skipping meals (especially breakfast) can slow your basal metabolic rate. Also, when you skip meals or go too long without eating, it's hard not to think about food a lot and to avoid overeating at the next meal. Because you're then so hungry, you're more likely to choose fatty, sugary foods.

- *Watching the fat intake.* Fat is a concentrated source of calories, so it's easy to hike up your caloric intake by eating just a small amount. It's important to get *some* fat each day (the equivalent of about one tablespoon), but most people consume much more than this. Limiting fat intake is probably the easiest and most efficient way of lowering caloric intake.

- *Using alcohol in small quantities, if at all.* Alcohol provides very little nutrition, but (depending upon what it's mixed with and how much you drink) it can add a whopping number of calories to your diet. Alcohol also lowers inhibitions, possibly encouraging excess eating. In fact, a significant portion of the obese population might be slimmer if they drank less. It's best and safest to drink in moderation, preferably wine instead of beer or distilled spirits. For most adults, that means up to two drinks a day for a man and one a day for a woman. Alcohol can trigger gout, a painful joint disease that is a well-known secondary risk factor for OA. If you have gout, eliminate alcohol from your diet.

- *Never counting calories or "dieting."* People who are successful at losing and maintaining their weight do not follow stringent "diets" or burden themselves with calorie counting. Strict diets and calorie counts are too restrictive and burdensome; they're quickly dropped in favor of a more tolerable way of living. It's a much better idea to adopt a flexible, easy-to-follow general food plan that includes all the kinds of foods that you need to maintain health while slimming.

- *Not weighing themselves more than once a week.* It's normal for body weight to fluctuate a few pounds during the course of a single day, mostly due to changes in water content. Those who weigh themselves daily (or worse yet, several times a day) may become obsessed with the numbers on the scale, panicked when there is a slight gain or overly confident when there is a loss. Don't let your eating be dictated by the scale.

- *Being content with their bodies and realistic about their goals.* If you're 5'9" and 325 pounds, getting down to 125 pounds shouldn't be your primary goal. Numerous studies have shown that if you're overweight or obese, losing just 10 percent of your excess weight can have a significant positive effect on your health. Set a realistic weight loss goal. Once you've achieved it, you'll feel like a success, not a failure, and you'll be ready to set a new goal and achieve that as well. Accept yourself as you are today, while working to improve (even just a little bit) every day from now on.

- *Being organized.* Successful weight managers prepare in advance for events by eating full, well-balanced meals at home and, if necessary, bringing their own food along. They are committed to their goals. They arrange their schedules so that they always have time for nutritious meals and their exercise sessions, the most important meeting of the day.

- *Understanding the reasons for their overeating and past failures.* People eat for many reasons besides physical hunger. Many of us use food to quell pain, to deal with stress or unhappiness, to ease boredom, or just because we like the oral stimulation. Once you figure out why you overeat, substitute another activity. For instance, during my breaks at work I used to slip something into my mouth to give myself a time out. Then I realized I wasn't really hungry when I did this—I was eating only because of feeling stressed. I decided to substitute a healthier behavior. I now throw darts at my dart board or visit with a colleague down the hall during my break time.

What Makes Up a Healthy Diet?

It's relatively easy to eat well enough to prevent a major vitamin or mineral deficiency disease such as beriberi or scurvy. But a minor deficiency of any nutrient can leave the body in a weakened state, more susceptible to disease, and less equipped to fight off invaders.

Your body needs many different nutrients to keep running in peak form, including protein, carbohydrates, fats, fiber, vitamins, minerals, and phytochemicals. These are found in different combinations and different amounts in various foods. If you continually eat the same foods over and over (even foods high in nutrients), you may be missing out on important building blocks for your health. Not only is variety the spice of life, it's the spark plug of health.

Stopping the Joint Busters

Researchers have consistently found that consuming a healthful, varied diet is one of the most important things we can do to safeguard our health. But exciting news for osteoarthritis sufferers is emerging from research concerning a special connection between food and the symptoms of osteoarthritis. We now know that certain foods can help stem the destruction of joints, while others may help to ease the pain. And as we'll see, for some people, certain foods can actually *worsen* joint symptoms.

Several theories attempt to explain why our joints deteriorate. One of them holds that unstable molecules called *free radicals* roam about the body attacking and destroying healthy tissue, including the tissue found in the joints.

Damage from excess free radicals is thought to be a major cause of many diseases, including cancer, heart disease, and aging and degenerative diseases. Osteoarthritis may be at least in part the result of free radical damage. To make matters worse, joint inflammation itself may trigger an even faster rate of new free radical formation. That's why prevention of free radical damage is a critical feature in treating and preventing osteoarthritis.[5]

Luckily, antioxidants are a major help in fighting free radicals. Where can you find antioxidants? They're as close as your refrigerator or your nearest bottle of vitamins. The antioxidants include vitamin A (or beta carotene and other carotenoids, which are the plant form of the vitamin), vitamin C, vitamin E, and the mineral selenium. An easy way to remember them is the acronym ACES. Foods that contain any of the four ACES are powerful weapons for combating free radicals and the havoc that they wreak.

It's always best to get your ACES from whole foods, rather than from supplements, for when they're in the foods the antioxidants are mixed in with other substances that can also be critical in disease prevention. Here are some good food sources of the ACES:

- *Vitamin A, beta carotene, and the carotenoids.* Researchers have discovered that the carotenoids (beta carotene, the plant form of vitamin A, is one of dozens) are very effective in fighting free radicals. Carotenoids are found mostly in yellow-orange fruits and vegetables such as apricots, sweet potatoes, pumpkin, carrots, cantaloupe and other melons, mangoes, papaya, peaches, and winter squash, as well as the dark green leafy vegetables such as broccoli, spinach, collard greens, parsley, and other leafy greens. If you cut open a fruit or vegetable and see color inside, chances are that it is a good source of carotenoids. You'll find vitamin A in liver, turkey, milk, eggs, and other foods of animal origin.

- *Vitamin C.* At least some of this antioxidant is found in every kind of fruit and vegetable; it's also found in fresh meat. Outstanding sources of vitamin C in fruit include cantaloupe, grapefruit, papaya, kiwi, oranges, mangoes, raspberries, pineapples, bananas, strawberries, and tomatoes. The vegetables highest in vitamin C include Brussels sprouts, collard greens, cabbage, asparagus, broccoli, potatoes, and red peppers. Vitamin C is heat sensitive, so to preserve the maximum amount possible, eat fruits and vegetables raw or only lightly cooked.

- *Vitamin E.* The primary sources of this antioxidant are nuts, seeds, whole grains, and vegetable oils such as sunflower and safflower oil. Good dietary sources include sunflower seeds, wheat germ, avocados, peaches, whole-grain breads and cereals, spinach, broccoli, asparagus, dried prunes, and peanut butter. The refined vegetable oils sold in your supermarket don't have much vitamin E (or other nutrients) left in them. Cold-pressed vegetable oils, sold in health-food stores, are much higher in natural vitamin E.

- *Selenium.* Besides protecting your cells from the toxic effects of free radicals by helping to recycle vitamin E in your body and make the antioxidant enzyme glutathione, selenium can help to keep the immune system functioning properly. You can find good amounts of selenium in swordfish, salmon, tuna, organ meats, cracked wheat bread, oatmeal, brown rice, sunflower seeds, oysters, and shrimp.

Do You Need Supplements?

It's always best to get the vitamins and minerals that your body needs from fresh, whole foods rather than from supplements. Unfortunately, that's not always possible—we can't or don't always eat as well as we should. More importantly, the amounts of the antioxidant vitamins and other nutrients that are most effective for helping osteoarthritis are larger than you can reasonably get just from your food. Your body uses up a lot of antioxidants in fighting off the extra free radicals caused by the inflammation of arthritis, so you need to be sure you're getting plenty of the ACES, especially vitamin C. To do that, you'll need supplements.

The daily dosages I generally recommend for antioxidant supplements are:

- Vitamin A: 5,000 IU
- Vitamin C: 250 to 1,000 mg
- Vitamin E: 100 to 400 IU
- Selenium: 55 to 200 mcg

In addition, I generally recommend adding the trace mineral boron to your daily supplements. Boron helps to keep calcium in your bones, which is important for maintaining joint health and keeping bones strong; some studies have shown that boron can have a beneficial effect on osteoarthritis.[6] In geographic areas where boron intakes are low, osteoarthritis incidence is high, and vice versa, although other factors could also be at work.[7] Good dietary sources of boron are fruits such as apples, pears, and grapes; leafy green vegetables, nuts, and beans are also good sources. For supplementation, the recommended dosage is 1 to 3 mg per day for adults.

Strengthening the Joints with Bioflavonoids

Bioflavonoids is a broad term for a very large group of thousands of substances found in virtually all plant foods; they're the natural chemicals that give these foods their characteristic colors and tastes. Among other things, bioflavonoids are essential for healthy capillary walls and the metabolism of vitamin C. Overall, bioflavonoids can help osteoarthritis sufferers by:

- Reinforcing the ability of collagen to form a strong matrix.
- Preventing free radical damage.

- Slowing the inflammation response.
- Preventing collagen from being destroyed when the cartilage tissue is inflamed.
- Hastening the healing of injury.

The foods with the greatest concentrations of bioflavonoids include green tea, berries, onions, citrus fruits, and fruits that contain a pit (such as cherries and plums). Other sources include all fresh fruits, fresh vegetables, seeds, and whole grains. As a general rule, the more deeply colored a fruit or vegetable is, the more assorted bioflavonoids it contains.

Bioflavonoid supplements are sold in pharmacies and health-food stores as citrus bioflavonoids, rutin, quercetin, lycopene, hesperidin, catechins, gingko biloba extracts, milk thistle seed extracts, proanthocyanidins, lutein, zeaxanthin, and many more. New bioflavonoids are discovered all the time.

Although some individual bioflavonoids have been shown to have specific beneficial effects (a diet high in lycopene has been associated with low rates of prostate cancer, for instance), there really hasn't been enough research to say that any one bioflavonoid helps arthritis. But since fruits, vegetables, and whole grains are crammed with all kinds of bioflavonoids, the best approach is to eat as many richly colored fruits and vegetables as possible. That way, if any of them do have a good effect, you'll be sure to get it!

If you do want to try bioflavonoid supplements, here are some suggestions and recommended daily doses:

- Proanthocyanidins (sold under the trade name Pycnogenol®), 30 to 100 mg
- Curcumin (found naturally in the spice turmeric), 100 to 500 mg
- Garlic, 100 to 500 mg
- Green tea extract, 300 mg
- Mixed bioflavonoids, 500 to 1,000 mg

Some daily multivitamin supplements now include bioflavonoids such as lutein—check the labels.

Controlling Inflammation Naturally

Inflammation can be the source of much pain and discomfort for the owner of an osteoarthritic joint, occurring most often in the more advanced cases. Inflammation is the body's natural response to tissue damage, or to overuse of a diseased joint. Although well-intentioned, the inflammation response is what may make your joints feel stiff, warm, swollen, and achy.

Inflammation is one of the ways the body protects itself after injury or disease. When tissue is damaged, the white blood cells race to the "scene of the crime" to remove the damaged cells and attack any infection. As part of the natural response, they produce substances called *prostaglandins* and *leukotrienes,* which in turn starts a cascade of biochemical reactions, including inflammation. The white blood cells also produce free radicals such as hydrogen peroxide as part of the inflammation cascade—and that can damage the cartilage.

In arthritis, the inflammation persists long after the original injury or illness is gone. Your diet can play in role in bringing the inflammation down. It's a little complex, but here's how it works:

Fatty acids in your diet can alter this inflammation response, either for the better or for the worse. That's because your body uses fatty acids to make the many different prostaglandins (short-lived substances that act a lot like hormones) that are part of the cascade. Some prostaglandins increase inflammation, while others are designed to reduce it. *Arachidonic acid* is the main food culprit when it comes to producing inflammatory prostaglandins. Originating almost entirely in animal products and saturated fats, it is a precursor to the "bad" kind of prostaglandins that produce inflammation as well as platelet stickiness, hardening of the arteries, heart disease, and strokes. Meat, poultry, dairy products (especially those containing saturated fat), and egg yolks all contain arachidonic acid. If you have osteoarthritis, eat these foods in moderation.

Alpha-linolenic acid (ALA), eicosapentaenoic acid (EPA), gamma-linolenic acid (GLA), and *linoleic acid* are fatty acids that are used to make anti-inflammatory prostaglandins. What this means is that to an extent you can decrease the swelling and pain in your joints by eating foods and taking supplements high in anti-inflammatory fatty acids.

The Inflammation Fighters

Let's take a look at the fatty acids that can *reduce* inflammation:

Alpha-linolenic acid (ALA), also called (for complicated reasons I won't go into) omega-3 fatty acid, is found in green vegetables and other foods of plant origin such as nuts, seeds, and whole grains. It can help block the production of pro-inflammatory prostaglandins and leukotrienes.

Gamma-linolenic acid (GLA), also called omega-6 fatty acid, is found in black currant oil, evening primrose oil, and borage seed oil. It's a precursor of the good anti-inflammatory prostaglandins, so the more you have of it, the more of these "good" prostaglandins your body can make. Since GLA isn't really found in high concentrations in foods we normally eat, you'll have to use supplements. The usual daily dose is 200 to 500 mg. Unfortunately, GLA can also *trigger* inflammation in some people, so be cautious if you decide to take try it. You may be able to avoid this by balancing your intake of omega-6 fatty acids with foods or supplements rich in omega-3 fatty acids (see below).

Linoleic acid is found in plant oils such as corn, soybean, sunflower, safflower, flaxseed, and other vegetable oils—but only if they're not heavily processed, as are the cheap vegetable oils sold in supermarkets. Linoleic acid helps the body increase its level of EPA, which in turn blocks the production of harmful prostaglandins.

Eicosapentaenoic acid (EPA), the best known of the omega-3 fatty acids, is found in marine plants and fish. EPA is actually made by algae, plankton, and seaweed, which are then eaten by certain fish. Not all fish are good sources of EPAs—freshwater fish have relatively little. Coldwater fatty fish caught in the ocean have the greatest amounts, including mackerel, anchovies, herring, salmon, sardines, Atlantic sturgeon, and tuna. Eating as little as one ounce of fish per day, or two fish meals a week, can help reduce inflammation. (Be aware that deep-frying destroys omega-3 fatty acids, besides adding loads of unhealthful fat.) There's a bonus to eating fish at least twice a week: you also reduce your risk of heart disease and diabetes.

Although it's always better to get your nutrients from real food, some people take their omega-3s in supplement form as fish oil capsules. The usual dose for helping arthritis inflammation is at least 1,000 mg daily and up to 5,000 mg per day for more severe cases. Be careful not to overdo either method of consumption, however, since too much fish or fish oil can interfere with your blood's ability to clot, especially if you also take drugs or supplements that thin your blood (aspirin, ginko biloba, high-dose vitamin E, and some prescription drugs). Excessive intake of fish oil capsules can lead to overdoses of vitamins A and D (especially if you're also getting these nutrients in your vitamin supplement), which can be toxic.

Food Allergies and Arthritis

It's possible that some of your arthritis symptoms are due to food allergies and intolerances—either acute or delayed onset—and that eliminating these foods from your diet will help your symptoms.

An *acute food allergy* is the result of an exaggerated immune system response to a food that your body mistakenly believes is harmful. Once your immune system labels a particular food as harmful, it creates specific antibodies to it. After that, each time your body see that same food, your immune system releases massive amounts of histamine, a chemical designed to protect the body. The histamine response can trigger a cascade of allergic symptoms that can cause sudden rashes, hives, welts, inflammation, and even anaphylactic shock (breathing difficulties, massive drops in blood pressure, and death without immediate medical treatment). This type of food reaction appears quickly, from a couple of minutes up to two hours after consuming the offending food.

Delayed onset food allergy (DOFA for short) is also known as food intolerance, food sensitivity, or food hypersensitivity. It's a slower reaction to some of the foods you eat—the symptoms build up over time. Delayed onset food allergies generally cause some form of inflammatory response or a variety of other symptoms such as chronic fatigue, joint and muscle pain, acne, eczema, headaches, mental "cloudiness," and a host of digestive disturbances, to name a few.

The problem with delayed onset food allergies is that they are hard to diagnose and often get mistaken for other health problems. For instance, if you have a slow reaction to a food, your body's response might be a flare-up of your joint pain several days after you eat it. You—and your doctor—might not connect something you ate on Monday with joint pain on Thursday. People who suffer from delayed onset food allergy usually have *more* than one symptom. In fact, it's unlikely that a person with just one symptom can blame delayed onset food allergy as the cause. So, if you have flare-ups of both joint pain *and* digestive problems, for instance, DOFA might be the underlying cause.

How Food Can Become the Enemy

Delayed onset food allergies occur when large molecules of food proteins enter the bloodstream and are circulated around the body. If you happen to be allergic to those particular food proteins, your immune system sees these proteins as invaders and attacks them.

In most cases, people develop delayed onset food allergy after being on antibiotics, especially when these drugs are taken over weeks or months. Prolonged use of anti-inflammatory drugs (both over-the-counter and prescription) or acid blockers, especially the "proton pump inhibitors" such as omeprazole (Prilosec®), lansoprazole (Prevacid®), and esomeprazole magnesium (Nexium®), seem to cause the problem in some as well. The theory is that these drugs may alter the populations of healthy bacteria normally present in the GI tract. In millions of people yearly, NSAIDs (even enteric-coated and COX-2 selective ones) cause erosions in the stomach lining, sometimes all the way down to the blood vessels. Without the protective lining intact, food proteins can just waltz directly into the bloodstream, bypassing the normal mechanism of stomach permeability and the proper immune reaction.

CELIAC SPRUE

Perhaps the prototype of disorders related to food, autoimmune disease, and arthritis is a condition known as celiac disease or celiac sprue. People with celiac disease can't break down and absorb gluten, a grain protein, properly. The condition is actually quite common and may affect as many as one in 200 people. When people with celiac disease eat foods containing gluten (found in wheat, barley, rye, oats, and some other grains), the protein damages the villi (tiny, fingerlike projections) in the small intestine. This can lead to serious intestinal inflammation and malnutrition, because nutrients can't be properly absorbed. The only current and effective treatment for celiac sprue is lifelong avoidance of any form of gluten in the diet. Unfortunately, that can be very difficult to do. In addition, people with celiac sprue also often have other food sensitivities. Because of poor nutrient absorption, celiac sprue sufferers often have significant joint problems that can go undiagnosed or misdiagnosed for a long period of time. Osteoporosis, weight loss, and bowel problems (such as chronic diarrhea) are also often present, and again, they can go on for a long time before the correct diagnosis is made.

Diagnosing DOFA

The delayed onset food allergy (DOFA) reaction generally kicks in anywhere from two to 72 hours after eating the reactive foods. The range of symptoms can affect any organ or tissue, and and there is often a slow, cumulative reaction over time. Due to the delay of the reaction, and because often four or five different foods can be implicated, identifying the offending foods is very difficult. Elimination and challenge diets are the gold standards in identifying the rogue foods, but these are very time-consuming and exhausting methods.

A faster method is the enzyme-linked immunosorbent assay (ELISA) laboratory test, which can provide a rapid and precise method of detecting the foods to which you have an immunoglobulin G (IgG) antibody reaction. (IgG is a substance produced by your body as part of the allergic response.) Since delayed onset food allergy often results in an immune reaction to food proteins over time, the body builds up higher levels of antibodies specifically to these foods. During the analysis, sophisticated instrumentation is used to measure the amount of food-specific IgG antibodies created within your blood. This method lets the lab identify which foods you have shown a strong reaction to (and therefore should avoid), those you have shown a moderate reaction to, and those you have shown no reaction to, so you can eat them freely.

When it comes to testing for food allergies, I have been very impressed by the accuracy and convenience of York Nutritional Laboratories (www.yorkallergyusa.com). Without the need for a doctor's visit, traditional blood draw, or trip in your car, the York blood test is the easiest and most cost-effective I know.

Food allergy tests have provided many thousands of people around the world with the health relief they have been looking for, often after many years of unsuccessful treatment for chronic illness through conventional methods. A simple dietary change is sometimes all that is needed to bring long-term symptomatic relief for many. I encourage all my patients with autoimmune diseases, including rheumatoid arthritis and lupus, to undergo this testing. For osteoarthritis sufferers, I usually recommend the test only if they have other vague symptoms, or if they suspect an aggravation of their arthritis some time after eating certain foods.

Putting It All Together: Eating to Beat Osteoarthritis

We've covered a lot of nutritional ground here. Now it's time to put it all together. The four elements of a powerful anti-osteoarthritis diet are foods filled with antioxidants, foods that contain bioflavonoids, foods that reduce inflammation, and foods that enable you to keep your weight under control. Let's see exactly what you can eat to incorporate into your diet these four ways to fight osteoarthritis.

OSTEOARTHRITIS FIGHTER 1 *Foods That Contain Antioxidants*

Vitamin A/carotenoids.   Yellow-orange fruits and vegetables such as apricots, sweet potatoes, pumpkin, carrots, cantaloupe, mangoes, papaya, peaches, and winter squash. Also dark green leafy vegetables such as broccoli, spinach, collard greens, parsley, and other leafy greens.

Vitamin C.   Cantaloupe, grapefruit, papaya, kiwi, oranges, mangoes, raspberries, pineapples, bananas, strawberries, tomatoes, brussels sprouts, collard greens, cabbage, asparagus, broccoli, potatoes, and red peppers.

Vitamin E.   Cold-pressed vegetable oils (sunflower and safflower), sunflower seeds, wheat germ, nuts, avocados, peaches, whole-grain breads and cereals, spinach, broccoli, asparagus, dried prunes, and peanut butter.

Selenium.   Swordfish, salmon, tuna, organ meats, cracked wheat bread, oatmeal, brown rice, sunflower seeds, oysters, and shrimp.

Summing Up #1: To Get Plenty of Antioxidants . . .

Eat at least one food from the vitamin A/carotenoids list and two from the vitamin C list daily. One tablespoon vegetable oil or one other food from the vitamin E list daily is sufficient. Eat one selenium-rich food and one boron-rich food per week.

If you wish to take supplements of the ACES, check with your doctor. Nutritionally minded physicians generally consider these to be safe ranges for most adults: vitamin A (5,000 IU); vitamin C (250 to 1,000 mg); vitamin E (100 to 400 IU), selenium (55 to 200 mcg), boron (1 to 3 mg).

OSTEOARTHRITIS FIGHTER 2 *Foods That Contain Bioflavonoids*

You'll find bioflavonoids in citrus fruits, berries, green tea, onions, fruits that contain a pit (such as cherries and plums), and whole grains. In general, plant foods that are richly colored are good sources of bioflavonoids. Eat at least one food rich in bioflavonoids per day.

OSTEOARTHRITIS FIGHTER 3 *Foods That Reduce Inflammation*

Omega-3 fatty acids. Omega-3s are the best natural inflammation fighters, and EPA, or fish oil, is the best of the omega-3s. The best dietary source is coldwater fish such as mackerel, anchovies, herring, salmon, sardines, Atlantic sturgeon, and tuna, all good sources of EPA. (But don't deep-fry them.) Eating two to five fish meals per week is recommended. If you don't eat fish you may want to take supplements of 1,000 to 2,000 mg of fish oil per day. Because fish oil can interfere with blood clotting, do not take more than 2,000 mg daily. Discuss fish oil with your doctor before trying it.

Evening primrose oil, black currant oil, and borage seed oil. These oils all contain gamma-linolenic acid (GLA), which is an acceptable (although less effective) substitute for EPA. However, GLA may trigger inflammation in some people, so use with caution. These oils will work with your diet, but they do tend to be expensive. A standard daily dose is about 500 mg.

Plant oils such as corn, soybean, sunflower, safflower, or flaxseed. These contain linoleic acid, which helps the body increase EPA levels and thus lessens the inflammatory response. One tablespoon per day (about 1,000 mg) should be helpful for most people.

Choose minimally refined, cold-pressed vegetable oils and store them in the refrigerator. Flaxseed oil also comes in capsules.

Summing Up #3: To Use Your Diet to Help Lessen the Inflammation Response . . .

Eat two to five fish meals per week; *or* take one to two tablespoons (1,000 to 2,000 mg) fish oil daily; *or* take about 500 milligrams of evening primrose oil, black currant oil, or borage seed oil; or take 1 tablespoon (1,000 mg) of the plant oils listed above.

OSTEOARTHRITIS FIGHTER   4 *Keep Your Weight under Control*

Follow the traditional Mediterranean diet when selecting foods and amounts for your basic eating plan. Take supplements as indicated. Concentrate on lower-fat, nutrient-rich foods and eating plenty of fresh fruits and vegetables. Substitute whole grains for white flour and limit potatoes, rice, and pasta. Do not skip meals or "diet" to lose weight. Put most of your time and energy into fitness, especially improving your aerobic capacity and strength. And remember to make changes gradually, sticking with them until they become second nature.

Arthritis Diet Myths

A good diet can help you control some of the symptoms of osteoarthritis, but there is no single diet that can "cure" arthritis. Beware of diets that require an excessive amount of one food or nutrient, or diets that require you to leave out entire food groups. And watch out for these three popular dietary myths:

- **Arthritis Diet Myth #1:** *Removing "nightshade" vegetables from your diet can relieve sore joints.* This myth emerged in the 1960s when a horticulturist from Rutgers University noticed that he personally experienced sore joints after eating nightshade vegetables. Nightshades come from the plant genus *Solanum* and include more than 1,700 herbs, shrubs, and trees, including eggplant, bell peppers, potatoes, and tomatoes. Although there are many claims that removing nightshades will cure arthritis, no scientific proof has been offered.
- **Arthritis Diet Myth #2:** *The Dong Diet can significantly improve the symptoms of arthritis.* The Dong Diet is an elimination diet developed by Collin Dong, M.D., patterned after the diet that many Chinese have followed for centuries. The diet calls for the elimination of all preservatives, additives, fruits, red meat, herbs, alcohol, and dairy products. There is absolutely no scientific proof that this diet works. Though this diet does not appear to be particularly unhealthy, any benefit felt by some people may well be due to eliminating foods that cause an immune reaction.
- **Arthritis Diet Myth #3:** *A "natural" diet rich in alfalfa can reduce the symptoms of arthritis.* There's no evidence that this works— and alfalfa taken in high doses can interfere with normal red blood cell production. A good diet needs to include a great deal more than just high amounts of a certain food.

Fad diets for osteoarthritis will always come and go, but when you look at them closely, the scientific basis is nonexistent or based on a distorted interpretation of a single small study. For the best results from the Arthritis Cure, stick to the safe and sound principles of a nutritious diet, keep your weight down, and consider using the supplements discussed in this chapter.

—10—

BEATING THE BLUES

What is depression?

*What is the link between depression
and osteoarthritis?*

What are the signs of depression?

Who is at risk for becoming depressed?

How can I beat the blues?

What are antidepressants?

*What is SAMe and how can it help depression
and osteoarthritis?*

What are "keeping up" and "covering up"?

How do stress and fatigue worsen depression?

*How can I make my body more stress- and
fatigue-resistant?*

How can I get a better night's sleep?

Robin's problem began very slowly. At first she simply slept a little later every morning and felt slightly fatigued when she woke up. But two years after it began, she was tired all the time. Routine chores exhausted her, and she had no energy for her husband or her friends. Thinking that it might be a problem with her endocrine system, her immune system, her nervous system, or her heart, a phalanx of doctors put her through a variety of tests and wound up prescribing "a bunch of medicines, I forgot how many." Of course, the drugs had side effects, including depression, so new drugs had to be used to quell the harmful effects of the old ones. The doctors never found anything to explain Robin's fatigue. The only thing wrong with this otherwise textbook-healthy 35-year-old woman was rather severe osteoarthritis of the right knee.

Osteoarthritis: That was the problem. Not directly, for osteoarthritis does not cause fatigue or emotional upset. But anything that produces pain, limits mobility, and threatens disability can lead to depression, which, in turn, can result in fatigue, listlessness, lack of interest in family and friends, sexual difficulties, and many other problems. It turns out that Robin had been a very promising fencer, possibly a candidate for the Olympics, when at age 23 osteoarthritis of her right knee, her "lunging knee," forced her to set aside her sword. All at once, her dreams were shattered and her future ripped away. She became depressed. And her unhappiness deepened as the pain in her knee grew, forcing her to give up the jogging and beach volleyball she had enjoyed with her husband and friends. "I felt old and used up at twenty-five," she sighed. "No wonder I was depressed."

Depression—persistent feelings of sadness, tiredness, low self-esteem, and lack of interest in daily activities and things you used to enjoy—is a common side effect of osteoarthritis. It's natural to be upset as pain forces you to give up your favorite activities, makes routine chores difficult, and reminds you of its presence even when you're sitting down. The risk of depression rises as the pain becomes more severe and the disability increases, with unpredictable pain flare-ups making you feel like a hostage to the disease. Indeed, some researchers believe that loss of function or disability is even more likely to induce depression than is pain.[1] About 20 percent of osteoarthritis sufferers are depressed at any given time, a percentage consistent with the level of depression found among other groups of people with chronic diseases.[2]

Depression is surprisingly common no matter what your age, sex, or level of health. According to the National Institute of Mental Health, nearly 19 million adult Americans, or about 9.5 percent of the adult population, have a depressive disorder in any given year. Nearly twice as many women (12.0 percent) as men (6.6 percent) are affected by a depressive disorder each year. That works out to 12.4 million women and 6.4 million men. Major depressive disorder is the leading cause of disability in the United States. Because of the treatment involved, and the missed work, the annual cost of depression is estimated between $44 and $53 billion.[3]

The magnitude of the importance and influence of depression in those affected by OA is exemplified by the following astounding fact: The presence and degree of depression is more correlated to the symptoms of OA pain than even that person's X rays![4] In other words, if you have OA, your level of pain can be predicted just by whether you're depressed, and if you are, by how severe your depression is.

Not everyone with arthritis gets depressed, but we know that any disease that causes constant pain often causes depression—even if it's mild and temporary—as well. There is plenty of good evidence to show that you need to treat depression to be actively involved in controlling your condition. People who use passive coping styles (resting, catastrophizing, and worrying) that are common in depression report higher levels of pain and disability in a number of chronic disorders, including arthritis.[5] This is why I strongly advocate following the entire treatment program in the arthritis cure, including the exercise part. It works much better than just sitting at home and taking pain pills, despite what you see in the commercials for arthritis drugs on television.

SAMe Benefits Depression and Osteoarthritis

SAMe occurs naturally in the body and is a cofactor in dozens of critical biochemical pathways. Research dating as far back as 1976 suggested that SAMe might be helpful for depression. SAMe had been found in various regions of the brain and it was known that certain psychiatric medications could increase the levels of SAMe in the bloodstream.

The first use of SAMe for treatment of depression led to some unexpected good fortune. Further investigation of SAMe showed that it had some anti-inflammatory and pain-relieving properties. Some of the patients in the research studies who had osteoarthritis along with depression reported a symptomatic benefit while using SAMe. This led to research on SAMe for osteoarthritis.

Initial research was limited to the prescription market, since SAMe could only be administered by injection. Research progressed when a stable form of SAMe that could be taken orally became available as a dietary supplement. Improvements in production over the years have made SAMe even more stable. Today high-quality SAMe supplements are widely available without a prescription.

When treating depression, sometimes it is helpful and even necessary to use medication in addition to the other treatments I describe later in this chapter. But since prescription antidepressant medications such as fluoxetine (Prozac®) and sertraline (Zoloft®) still have a stigma among some people, and because the medications can have some significant side effects, people often look to alternatives. SAMe is one such alternative. A viable treatment for mild to moderate (but not severe) depression, SAMe has been found to be equally as effective as prescription antidepressants when studied head to head—and it doesn't have the side effects such as rashes, weight gain, loss of libido, and nausea often found with these drugs.

In 2002 researchers at the U.S. Agency for Healthcare Research and Quality (AHRQ), a division of the Department of Health and Human Services, performed a comprehensive review of 99 studies of SAMe.[6] In order to pull together the data from all the studies, the researchers had to find studies that were of similar design. Many of the studies were very small, with only a limited number of subjects under investigation, and couldn't really be used as part of the larger analysis. In the end, the researchers reviewed, combined, and analyzed the data on 28 studies that focus on SAMe and depression, 10 studies on SAMe and osteoarthritis, and 6 studies on SAMe and liver disease.

Overall, the results were positive. In treating depression, SAMe was able to show a similar outcome to conventional antidepressants, significantly lowering the Hamilton rating score for depression after treatment, compared to pretreatment levels. Unfortunately, there were not enough studies to compare SAMe to placebo, though the trend here was still in favor of SAMe.

Related to osteoarthritis, SAMe was shown to have an equivalent effect on relieving pain and improving function compared to NSAIDs. In determining how impressive a substance performs for treating the symptoms of osteoarthritis, researchers rank the outcome according to something called "the effect size." An effect size of zero means that the substance does not improve the symptoms at all. An effect size of 1.0 is equivalent to someone with severe osteoarthritis who has a joint replacement and becomes completely pain free afterward. The effect size comparing SAMe to NSAIDs was low but positive, coming in at 0.11. Compared to placebo, SAMe scored an effect size of 0.20 (low to moderate) for treating osteoarthritis.

It's important to note that the oral dosage of SAMe used in these clinical studies ranged from 400 mg to 1,600 mg per day (and higher for liver disease). Most of the studies on depression or OA used 800 mg or more per day. It's not likely that someone with arthritis would experience this same level of relief on a much lower dosage, though there are people who swear they notice an effect even at 400 mg per day.

To get an idea of how SAMe compares to glucosamine and chondroitin in relation to improving pain and function, we need only look at a review study published in the prestigious *Journal of the American Medical Association* in 2000.[7] Six double-blind and placebo-controlled studies (the "gold standard" for scientific studies) on glucosamine yielded an effect size of 0.44 (medium effect). Nine such studies on chondroitin scored an effect size of 0.78 (high effect). (Check back to chapters 3 and 4 for a full description of studies on glucosamine, chondroitin, and ASU.) As we saw above, SAMe has a low effect size of only 0.11.

So what does all this tell us about SAMe? First, because SAMe was able to treat mild to moderate depression as well as standard prescription antidepressant drugs, but without the significant side effects, we should really start to consider using SAMe as a treatment for depression. If used under a physician's supervision, SAMe would perhaps be the first line of attack for mild to moderate depression, prior to moving on to the conventional depression medications if needed. Bear in mind that we are not talking about using SAMe for severe or life-threatening depression. In these instances, there is no substitute for careful physician intervention and medication treatment as appropriate.

The second thing we gather from the studies on SAMe is that it does have some mild effect on improving the pain and function in osteoarthritis sufferers. Since it is not as powerful as the mainstays for improving joint health and OA, namely glucosamine, chondroitin, and ASU, perhaps SAMe should be considered as something that could be added if needed.

Certainly if someone is suffering from both osteoarthritis and depression, which is relatively common, then SAMe might be a good choice to use along with the mainstay joint-health supplements. SAMe is on the expensive side, however, and the cost for using the dosages utilized in the research is quite high. In my experience, however, many patients do well on a lower dosage of 400 mg, which cuts the cost somewhat.

High-quality SAMe costs about three to five times as much as glucosamine/chondroitin. I am very concerned about the quality of many of the SAMe products available in the marketplace. When a supplement ingredient is very expensive, manufacturers can be tempted to cut corners. Some of the manufacturers of products on the market today are not careful in ensuring the stability and potency of the SAMe and some of the products use a form of SAMe that is only half as effective as the form used in the research. To help you choose a quality product, I've provided a list on my Web site at www.drtheo.com.

What Is—and Is Not—Depression?

We commonly use the word *depression* to describe a large group of emotional disorders, ranging from mild to severe, that occur on a chronic, recurrent, or one-time-only basis.

Chronic depressive disorders may last for years or even decades, often with the symptoms striking most severely in the first two years. Recurrent depressive disorders will appear and disappear periodically, leaving the sufferer feeling healthy between episodes. And one-time-only bouts of depression may last for a just a few days or weeks, then vanish forever. If your doctor says that your depression is "clinical," it means that your symptoms are serious enough or frequent enough to warrant medical attention. "Subclinical" depression is a less severe version of the problem in which some symptoms are present, but they are not serious enough to lead to diagnosis or treatment, because the sufferer can still get by in his or her daily activities. If the number of subclinical symptoms increases or if they become more severe, however, treatment may be warranted.[8]

Then there's the blues, otherwise known as "the blahs" or "feeling down in the dumps." This is not true depression. Instead, it's usually a reaction to an unpleasant event such as losing a job or failing a test. We feel bad for a while, then bounce back to our normal emotional states. Reacting to negative or stressful situations with the blues is perfectly normal. In fact, it's healthy. It only becomes a serious problem if it lasts for a significant period of time, if it is out of proportion to the unhappy situation, or if you feel you cannot shake the feeling on your own.

The Signs of Depression

We all sometimes have mild symptoms of depression. It's only when the symptoms don't seem to go away, if they get worse, or if more symptoms appear, that you truly can be said to be depressed. If one or more of the symptoms on the list below lingers for weeks on end or longer, you may want to discuss the situation with your doctor:[9]

- loss of interest in the things you normally enjoy
- feelings of hopelessness
- feelings of anxiety
- low self-esteem
- lack of interest in sex
- irritability or blue moods
- restlessness or a slowed-down feeling
- feelings of worthlessness or guilt
- appetite changes leading to weight gain or loss
- constant lack of energy
- suicidal thoughts or thoughts of dying
- problems with concentration, thinking, or memory
- difficulty making decisions

- lack of sleep, or sleeping too much
- nightmares, especially with themes of loss, pain, or death
- headaches not caused by any other disease or condition
- digestive problems unrelated to any other disease or condition
- aches and pains not caused by any other disease or condition
- preoccupation or obsession with failure, illness, or other unpleasant themes
- fear of being alone

A sense that all the interest and enjoyment has gone out of life is a very typical symptom of depression. Constantly feeling tired and sleep disturbances are another. An ongoing loss of interest in sex is an easy-to-spot symptom of depression among those who had previously enjoyed healthy sex lives. Pain, depression, fatigue, and stress can wreak havoc on your sex life, increasing your depression and feelings of hopelessness.

These are not the only symptoms of depression, and having one or more of them does not necessarily mean that you are clinically depressed, but they can point to problem areas. Your emotional health is just as important as your physical health, so contact your doctor when you need help. (Don't use these guidelines for the purpose of self-diagnosis—only licensed and trained medical professionals are qualified to render a diagnosis.)

Who Is Most Likely to Become Depressed?

Doctors and psychologists have identified specific risk factors that increase the odds of depression. These apply to the general population, not just osteoarthritis sufferers. Your risk is increased if:[10]

- You are a woman.
- You have already experienced a depressive event.
- Your first depressive event happened before age 40.
- You have a chronic medical condition or disease (including debilitating osteoarthritis).
- You have just had a baby.

- You have little or no emotional support (such as family and friends).
- You have just experienced a positive or negative stressful life event.
- You abuse drugs or alcohol.
- Your family has a history of depressive disorders.
- Earlier depressive events have only been partially relieved.
- You have attempted suicide.

You are not doomed to depression if you have one or more of these risk factors, and you are not guaranteed a depression-free life if you don't. However, this list of risk factors helps identify those who may be more susceptible to depression so they, their families, and physicians can watch for early signs of possible trouble.

Keeping Up and Covering Up

People with osteoarthritis often develop a variety of techniques to help them maintain their daily activities despite chronic pain. "Keeping up" occurs when you continue at your previous level of activity, despite increased pain or injury. You "keep up" because you want to prove that everything is okay. You may continue playing basketball on the weekends, or refuse work modifications that might make your job more manageable. It's possible for many people to "keep up" during the day, although they often suffer from excruciating pain and fatigue all evening and at night.

"Covering up" is an attempt to hide the osteoarthritis. You'll claim that you feel fine when people ask, even when you hurt. You'll refuse to use a cane, walker, or other device to assist you, because to do so would require you to acknowledge the pain. Instead of letting others see that you hurt, you may withdraw.

When "keeping up" or "covering up," you unwittingly cut off helpful support from your friends and loved ones, just when you need it most. This can cause strains among your family and friends, and it can contribute to depression.

Help for Depression

If you have any sense that you may be depressed, get professional help immediately. Ask your doctor for a referral to a therapist—he or she will want you to find the help you need. If you don't feel comfortable asking for help from your doctor, ask a trusted friend or other health professional, such as a nurse, for a referral. Today most people—and certainly most health professionals—understand that depression is a common and treatable problem. There's no need to feel ashamed or embarrassed if you decide you need to seek professional help.

Before your medical doctor refers you to a therapist, she or he should rule out the possibility of the depression being caused by a hormonal imbalance, Parkinson's disease, Huntington's disease, chronic fatigue syndrome, severe vitamin deficiency, or other ailments. And since some commonly prescribed drugs can cause depression, your doctor should also ask you what medications you are currently or have recently been taking. If physical causes for your depression have been ruled out, you may need the help of a mental health professional.

Therapy can be expensive, and it's not always fully covered by health insurance. If you can't afford to pay for therapy, however, you still have many options. Start with your local mental health department—you may qualify for reduced-rate programs. You can also check with local and state professional mental health organizations, osteoarthritis self-help groups, or your local chapter of the Arthritis Foundation.

If Your Osteoarthritis Has Left You Depressed . . .

Keep reminding yourself that your symptoms of depression will most likely improve or even vanish once the Arthritis Cure eliminates your pain and allows you to return to a normal life. In the meantime . . .

Psychotherapy (the "talking cure") and drug therapy are the two major approaches to treating depression. Mild to moderate episodes of depression are usually treated with counseling methods such as psychotherapy or cognitive/behavioral therapy (CBT—I'll talk more about this very helpful form of therapy later in this chapter). In severe cases, drug therapy with antidepressant is often started immediately. The combined approach—psychotherapy or CBT and drug therapy— is becoming a popular treatment for most episodes of depression, even mild ones. The combined approach is being used more for several reasons.

First, it helps reestablish normal body patterns more quickly. Antidepressants can be used to normalize many of the problem areas affected by depression: sleep, appetite, sexual desire, and energy level. The sooner these areas return to normal states, the quicker the individual is on the road to full recovery.

Combined therapy also helps to ensure compliance in taking medications. Doctors know that patients receiving help from psychotherapy are much more likely to take their medicines than those who do not have the additional support.

Finally, combined therapy recognizes the dual influence of biology and environment in causing depression. When researchers used PET (positron emission tomography) scans to create images of the brains of mentally ill patients, they observed that the use of medication and the use of psychotherapy separately created identical changes in brain activity. In other words, psychotherapy and drug therapy influence the brain in similar ways. Using the two together is believed to be stronger than either one alone.

Unfortunately, a lot of the standard medications used for osteo-arthritis can cause depression—even if you've never been depressed before. Prednisone, indomethacin, and other painkillers used for osteoarthritis are well known to cause depression in some patients. So can certain tranquilizers, including "downers" such as diazepam (Valium®, Ativan®) and chlordiazepoxide (Librium®). Codeine and other painkillers may cause or add to an existing depressive state. Sleeping pills may contribute to depression by altering your sleep patterns. That's why it's important to talk with your doctor before taking any medications—and why it's important to use nondrug methods as much as possible for improving your arthritis symptoms.

Common Antidepressive Medicines

Depression is a complex, mysterious syndrome, which is why developing medications to relieve its symptoms has been a complicated procedure. Today's antidepressant medications include several classes of drugs that can change the chemical activity of the brain. Each group of drugs has differing effects on brain chemistry, which present a challenge to doctors prescribing them. Perhaps the biggest problem with antidepressants is their side effects, which can include dry mouth, nausea, diarrhea, headache, insomnia, jitteriness, dizziness, constipation, increased perspiration, appetite stimulation, anorexia, confusion, impotence and delayed orgasm, and, in men over 50, difficulty urinating. More severe complications include elevated blood pressure, irregular heartbeat, tremors, nausea, stroke, and anxiety. An overdose can lead to toxicity and possibly death.

Antidepressants also take a long time to work. Two, four, or up to eight weeks may pass before any positive changes are seen. And the initial improvements may be very subtle—a slightly more erect posture, smiling a little bit more, taking a little extra care about one's appearance. The patient's family often notices the changes before the patient does.[11]

Although medicines certainly have their place in treating depression, sometimes they just mask the symptoms, ignoring the underlying causes. And their side effects can be more unpleasant and dangerous than the original problem. Glucosamine, ASU, and chondroitin, on the other hand, can be powerful "antidepressants," not because they work directly on your mood, but because they help eliminate the underlying problem. There's no such thing as an overnight miracle, though; it takes time for these two healing substances to work. That's why it's important to use a variety of depression-busting techniques. Some are stronger, some work faster, others last longer. Together, they can help to ensure recovery. And remember: If you are depressed because of osteoarthritis, your depression will likely clear up once the Arthritis Cure has gone to work.

Cognitive/Behavioral Therapy

Often people who are mildly or moderately depressed, stressed out, or anxious don't need to be treated by lengthy psychoanalysis. Many people benefit greatly from a form of psychotherapy called cognitive/behavioral therapy (CBT), a treatment based on the idea that it is our way of thinking that causes us to feel and act the way we do. By helping you understand how the way you think influences the way you feel and act, CBT helps you change unwanted feelings and behavior. CBT is goal oriented and fairly short term. Most patients achieve good results in less than 20 sessions. CBT is often drug-free, although people who find antidepressant drugs helpful can certainly still benefit from the therapy while continuing to take the drugs.

The goal of CBT is to give patients more control over their lives and to help them achieve specific goals, such as being able to cope better with a medical problem or feel less anxious. The philosophy behind CBT is that most emotional and behavioral responses are learned—and that means that with the help of a trained therapist you can unlearn the unwanted responses and learn new ones instead. To get the most from CBT, you'll have to do some homework—reading assignments and practicing some of the techniques you're taught—but the work usually pays off in better coping skills and less anxiety and depression.

To find a trained CBT therapist near you, contact either of these two professional organizations:

National Association of Cognitive-Behavioral Therapists
102 Gilson Avenue
Weirton, WA 26062
800-853-1135
www.nacbt.org

Association for Advancement of Behavior Therapy
305 Seventh Avenue
New York, NY 10001
212-647-1890
www.aabt.org

Coping with Depression

If you become depressed because of restrictions osteoarthritis has placed on your life, learning how to cope will do a lot of make you feel better. Mental health experts agree that those who cope best with disease are least likely to develop depression.[12] In other words, if you deal with your osteoarthritis in a positive and constructive way, it's less likely to leave you depressed.

Some of the best coping techniques are problem-solving and flexibility. People who tackle their problems head-on, coming up with creative solutions, do better. So do those who bend with the changes in their lives, adopting new activities, approaches, and ideas as they are forced to lay aside the old. For example, a creative, flexible person with osteoarthritis of the knee who can no longer jog for exercise may switch to swimming. Someone who lacks those coping skills may just decide to stop exercising and watch TV instead—which will only make the arthritis worse and could lead to depression.

Cognitive/behavioral therapy can help you learn better coping skills, but not everyone needs that level of assistance. Whether or not you decide to seek the help of a therapist, joining an arthritis support group where you can find sympathetic ears and get some advice on coping is also a good idea. Each support group has a different tone, depending on the leader and the participants. If you feel a particular group is spending too much time moaning and complaining, find one that emphasizes overcoming problems and getting on with your life. Support groups for arthritis (and many other chronic problems) are available almost everywhere. There's usually little or no cost. You can find self-help groups in your area by contacting the Arthritis Foundation, calling your local hospital, or asking your doctor.

Beating Stress Helps Beat Depression

If osteoarthritis has made you depressed, take care to avoid as much stress as possible until you're feeling better, physically and emotionally. Stress is the response of the body, mind, and emotions to both the everyday and extraordinary pressures of life. Stress is not the actual thing or event—it's our reaction. For example, being laid off from work may devastate one person, while another may find it an opportunity to find a better job or retire early. The situation is the same; it's the reaction that differs.

The fact that stress is the reaction, not the event itself, helps explain why some people are more stressed by their osteoarthritis than others. Some don't let their pain and disability bother them as much as others do. But even among those who take it relatively well, osteoarthritis can be a stressful event. Stress hits us in different ways, with symptoms that include:

- fatigue
- muscle tension
- anxiety
- irritability and anger
- upset stomach
- nervousness, trembling
- cold, sweaty hands
- loss or increase in appetite
- overall malaise (weakness, dizziness, headache, back pain, and other problems with no physical cause)

Anxiety—feelings of fear, apprehension, and tension—is a common response to stress. Developing arthritis is certainly a stressful situation, so it's not surprising that some people with arthritis experience anxiety and a sense of helplessness. High levels of anxiety are associated with high levels of disability from arthritis. In one recent study of patients with knee arthritis, for instance, the patients who felt the most anxiety had the highest levels of pain and disability, no matter how much joint damage was visible on their X rays.[13] Other studies have also shown that psychological factors, such as feelings of helplessness and anxiety, play a role in how much pain you feel from an arthritic joint.[14]

Stress and anxiety may not cause depression, but they can certainly make it worse (you've probably noticed that some of the stress symptoms we've listed here are very similar to the symptoms of depression). Stress also signals certain glands, such as your adrenal glands, to release high-voltage hormones that can "shock" the body and weaken the immune system, making your osteoarthritis symptoms seem worse while increasing your risk of getting another disease.

The best defense against stress is a positive attitude. Remember, stress is not the event or thing—that's just the stressor. How you respond to the stressor determines whether or not you're stressed. This means that you can literally "think" stress away. Please understand: You are not responsible for being stressed; it's not your fault. However, by focusing on the problem in a positive way, you can handle the stress. The good news is that by focusing on all that is pleasant, optimistic, loving, helpful, and joyful in your life, even if there are also sad or unpleasant things happening, you can take a big bite out of stress. The unhappy event (your osteoarthritis) will still be there, but your reaction to it will be different. Sure, arthritis is a pain. But is it worth getting unduly upset about, if doing so makes it worse? And yes, it's hard to smile in the face of adversity. But if smiling makes it better, then isn't smiling a medicine? That's why your prescription is to keep smiling, to fill your mind with thoughts of love, joy, and optimism. And while you're beating stress with a smile, you can also build yourself up physically.

Exercise regularly. Almost everyone can do some exercise, even those with severe osteoarthritis. If you can't jog anymore, try swimming. If aerobics class is too tough on your lower-body joints, try water aerobics or riding a stationary bike. Even if you're confined to bed, you can do strengthening exercises like leg lifts and upper-body work. Talk to your doctor or physical therapist about special exercises and activities that will help you maintain good posture and reduce stress on your joints.

Eat a healthful diet that gives your body all the nutrients it needs. Avoid sugar and caffeine, and stay away from fat- and sugar-laden fast foods and desserts. Eat plenty of nutrient-rich fresh vegetables and fruits, plus whole grains. If you drink alcoholic beverages, do so in moderation. Stay away from drugs unless they have been prescribed by your physician.

- Get plenty of sleep.
- Find a relaxation technique such as yoga or meditation that works for you and practice it daily.
- Think of a way you can change your life for the better, then make that change.
- Learn to balance rest and activity—in other words, pace yourself.
- When you have an arthritis flare-up, modify your activities and take more time to rest.
- Don't overextend yourself, and plan ahead for a difficult task.
- Ask for help when you need it.
- Limit your activities and responsibilities to manageable levels.

Get a Good Night's Sleep

One of the best defenses against stress, fatigue, and depression (unless your depression has prompted you to sleep too much) is getting a good night's sleep. When that happens, you wake up feeling refreshed and energetic, and the problems of yesterday and today don't seem as overwhelming. Here are some tips for better sleeping:

- Stick to a regular schedule of daily activity. Get up and go to bed at about the same time each day.
- Exercise regularly, but not late at night.
- Create a quiet and comfortable environment in which to sleep. Get heavy curtains to block out light if it bothers you. If you're sensitive to noise, try a "white noise" machine that covers outside noises with the soothing sounds of a waterfall or waves on the beach.
- Spend an hour winding down with a book or some other quiet activity before going to bed.
- Take a relaxing bath before going to bed.
- Practice relaxation techniques.
- Listen to soothing music.
- Avoid caffeine in the evening.

• Beware of alcohol. A nightcap before bed can actually leave you feeling tired and unrested in the morning.

Get Touched

Touch is a powerful healing tool—its health-giving properties have been demonstrated over and over. Take newborn babies, for example. Studies comparing premature babies who are not touched with those who are gently touched have found that the "touched" babies gained 45 to 50 percent more weight while in the hospital. The "touched" babies were more alert, active, and involved in their surroundings, and they went home earlier. The effects were lasting, for the "touched" babies tended to have fewer medical problems later in their young lives.[15] Adults also benefit from being touched. Many medical scientists believe that touch can reduce psychological stress. And only a very soft touch is required—bear hugs are not a necessity. In fact, a bear hug may be too much for many osteoarthritis sufferers! A gentle, loving touch is a powerful medicine for everyone, one that can be very beneficial in fighting arthritis.

You Can Overcome Depression

Osteoarthritis can produce a host of psychological changes due to pain, frustration, depression, and stress. The Arthritis Cure tackles depression in two ways. First, glucosamine/chondroitin and ASU help by attacking the problem at the source—the osteoarthritis itself. Second, it gives you healthy mind and body techniques that are known to beat the blues. This two-pronged approach will help you overcome depression while regaining your emotional and physical health.

—11—

YOU CAN PREVENT OSTEOARTHRITIS

This chapter will introduce you to the 8-step Osteoarthritis Prevention Program:

1. Prevent joint injuries.

2. Ensure proper recovery if you are injured.

3. Eat a healthful, joint-preserving diet.

4. Maintain your ideal weight.

5. Exercise regularly.

6. Optimize your biomechanics to counteract stress to your joints.

7. Consider preventive use of glucosamine/chondroitin and ASU

8. Use joint-supporting dietary supplements.

It's nice to know that the Arthritis Cure, spearheaded by glucosamine/chondroitin and ASU, can treat osteoarthritis once it has struck. But wouldn't it be even better to prevent the painful problem from rearing its ugly head in the first place?

We can. The 8-step Osteoarthritis Prevention Program can dramatically lower the risk of healthy joints suffering from osteoarthritic degeneration. It's impossible to absolutely guarantee that you will never be stricken by osteoarthritis, but we do know that the preventive program can work wonders. If you're reading this book, you probably already have osteoarthritis in at least one joint. You certainly don't want the other joints to suffer, so follow the prevention program to keep your other joints healthy, mobile, and pain-free. Once again, consult with your doctor before beginning this program.

You don't need high-tech medical instruments, highly paid specialists, exotic tests, or any other special tools to put the Osteoarthritis Prevention Program into action. All you need is some knowledge, a bit of time and thought, and determination to keep your joints healthy and strong. The prevention program is simple:

1. Prevent joint injuries.
2. Ensure proper recovery if you are injured.
3. Eat a healthful, joint-preserving diet.
4. Maintain your ideal weight.
5. Exercise regularly.
6. Optimize your biomechanics to counteract stress to your joints.
7. Consider preventive use of glucosamine/chondroitin and ASU.
8. Use joint-supporting dietary supplements.

That's all there is to it! And there are some great "side effects" to this program. By following the steps, you may also reduce your risk of having a heart attack or stroke and of developing cancer and many other serious diseases. You'll be putting yourself on the road to lifelong *great* health as you work to keep your joints strong and prevent ailments associated with painful joints.

Let's take a look at each of the eight points.

STEP 1 *Prevent Injuries*

Arthritis prevention really begins in childhood. It may be a little late in your life to be learning this, but my hope is that if you understand how to prevent arthritis perhaps you can help your children and grandchildren avoid it.

A child born today can expect to live about 80 years—if there aren't any dramatic breakthroughs in life-extending biotechnology. I believe there will be, however, because the medical technology is improving at an exponential rate. Life expectancy for a child born today could easily be 90 or even 100 years.

That's a far cry from life expectancy in 1900, when the average individual lived only 46 years. Since the majority of people start to feel the symptoms of osteoarthritis in their 40s or 50s, the average person suffering from osteoarthritis 100 years ago didn't suffer for very long. By the 1950s, life expectancy was about 60 years or more, and the incidence and prevalence of osteoarthritis was lower than that we have today. Even 50 years ago, people didn't have too many years of disability from their osteoarthritis.

Today's situation is quite different. With life expectancy approaching 80 years, and with future generations possibly living even longer, the average adult can expect to spend many years living with arthritis.

Age alone isn't the only arthritis risk factor that's increasing. Obesity and diabetes, both significant risk factors, are skyrocketing—not only among adults but among children as well. Obesity is now so common among children that an estimated one in three will develop Type 2 (adult-onset) diabetes in later life. While all too many kids and young adults today get little exercise, among those that play sports, injuries to the joints have increased. The frequency and intensity of practice and games in childhood athletics have increased steadily, and so have the injuries. Among the athletically talented, many dream of turning pro and making vast amounts of money—only to have their hopes cut short by serious joint injuries.

Title IX, the federal law that gives women an equal chance in school and college sports, has been great for increasing participation—but an increased injury rate came along for the ride. In many cases, rates of severe injury are higher for women than men playing the same sport, especially in basketball, volleyball, and soccer. In these sports, tears of the anterior cruciate ligament (ACL), the main stabilizing ligament in the knee, are several times more common in women than in men. ACL tears, and the resulting knee laxity often leads to early osteoarthritis. In fact, the way we study osteoarthritis in animals is by destabilizing the ACL. Unfortunately, it's not really known if attempts at surgical reconstruction of the ACL can really prevent osteoarthritis down the line. This makes it much more important to *prevent* the injury in the first place. I'm developing a program with the University of Arizona athletics department to try to reduce the incidence of ACL injuries. There are about 80,000 severe ACL injuries per year in the United States, a number that's just too high. Female soccer players in their teenage years who suffer an injury to the ACL frequently have X-ray diagnosable osteoarthritis by age 30, with 34 percent reporting some disability as a result. This percentage climbs as they age. If these women live to be 100, they may have disability for a full 70 years, something unheard of in human history.

Even with the dramatic breakthroughs detailed in this book, joint injuries can create a pathway to arthritis disability. We need to think now about how people will be able to keep their joints intact for 60, 70, and even 80 years into the future. The awareness needs to start in the young and with their parents. The interventions and preventive strate-gies I discuss in this chapter will help keep your joints in good shape as you age.

Injuries are a common cause of *secondary osteoarthritis*. So whether you're an occasional exerciser, a dedicated athlete, or anything in between, take special care of injuries to your joints and elsewhere. Sports that require pivoting, twisting, turning, and torqueing into unnatural positions (such as soccer, football, skiing, basketball, volley-ball, and tennis) are especially hard on the joints.

Fortunately, many sports-related joint problems can be avoided if you take simple precautions. Start by getting and staying in good con-dition. Train before you play, and consider getting professional coach-ing advice. Before hitting the slopes or stepping out on the tennis court, for example, exercise to build muscle strength around your joints and make your ligaments and tendons more resilient. Lifting weights three times a week during the "preseason" and at least once or twice a week when you're most active will help you keep up your strength. Doing sport-specific drills is even better. Go beyond just endurance and side-to-side drills and try moving in all directions against resis-tance, either from rubber tubing or from a stack of weights connected to a cable machine. Stretch often, but only after you've warmed up. And be sure to balance your exercise program. Don't focus on just one group of muscles to the exclusion of others, for that can cause more problems later on.

Be sure to use the proper shoes and other equipment (pads, eye protection, helmets, and so on). The proper shoes absorb shock, support your arches, and prevent you from sliding while you play (which can put extra stress on the joints). Your shoes should correspond to the playing surface, so wear running shoes while running, tennis shoes for tennis, and so forth. Replace your shoes often—worn-out shoes don't give you enough support or shock resistance.

Don't jump right into a high-level exercise program. Attempting to exercise like an Olympic athlete right off the bat can lead to injuries and frustration. Begin slowly; gradually increase the level of difficulty/proficiency and the amount of time you spend exercising. If you wish to run, for example, it might be wise to start with brisk walking, followed by jogging several weeks later and eventually running (when you're in better shape). Doing drills specific to your sport is a great way to prevent injury. This prepares the body for the unpredictability of movements needed in play.

Warm up before you get out and do *anything*. A short, brisk walk, five minutes on a stationary bike, or perhaps some jumping jacks and push-ups will help loosen your muscles and get the blood flowing.

Be sure to cool down and stretch after every exercise session. Once your muscles have been warmed up, they should be amenable to stretching—this is really the best time to increase your flexibility. Work on stretching several parts of your body, not just the muscles you use for your sport or exercise. And remember: Avoid stretching a "cold" muscle. That not only invites injury, it doesn't usually lead to any flexibility improvements.

Finally, get some training before you begin your new exercise or activity regimen. Don't just slap on the pads and start throwing body blocks; don't slide headfirst into home plate; don't put on the gloves and step into the boxing ring until you've learned exactly how it should be done. Even seemingly gentle sports, like swimming and bicycling, should be done properly in order to avoid injury. Technique is critical. You want to play your sport in a way that will let you enjoy it for years to come.

Sacrificing Your Body

Not so long ago, people played sports solely for the love of them. Professional athletes didn't make the incredible amounts of money they do today. Now that professional athletes have been elevated from players to celebrities with multimillion-dollar paychecks, aspiring athletes are willing to sacrifice their bodies and do anything, at any cost, to become successful. The tremendous incidence of performance-enhancing drug use among amateur and competitive athletes proves this point. Hundreds and hundreds of athletes die or have permanent organ damage every year from using drugs to try to increase their performance by just a few percentage points or fractions of a second.

The training and competition leading up to the big leagues lead to a lot of pressure to continue in the sport even after significant injury and subsequent surgeries. This doesn't come without a cost. Almost all professional athletes pay the arthritis price later for their days in the spotlight.

So many aging baby-boomer athletes and weekend warriors develop serious joint injuries that I have developed a special program at Canyon Ranch Resort to teach them what they can do to improve performance and increase their longevity in the sports they love. (More information is available at www.canyonranch.com.) In my experience there as a physician specializing in preventive medicine, most people don't see the medium- to long-range outcome of their decisions. Sometimes it takes me hours to get patients to understand that they need to vary their athletic activities to avoid joint damage, and that if injured they need to take the time to heal and rehabilitate properly. Going back to a sport too soon after an injury may let you play for a year or two more, but if you take the time to improve your strength, flexibility, technique, and biomechanics, you may be able to play happily for 20 or 30 more years.

Accidents and Arthritis

Sports participation is far from the only cause of injuries that lead to osteoarthritis in later life. Almost any significant injury can have this effect. There are hundreds of thousands of motor vehicle accidents each year in United States. Many of the collisions are minor, but even so, many result in damage to the joints. One condition is so common that it has its own name, "dashboard knee." As the occupant of the vehicle moves forward upon collision, the knees impact the dashboard, damaging the cartilage under the kneecap (and sometimes in the hip and lower back). This is a very common cause of osteoarthritis, but unfortunately the symptoms often don't show up until months or even a few years later. By that time, the victims have sometimes signed away their rights to obtain medical care related to the injury, even though they may be disabled for years.

Another common injury that leads to osteoarthritis is falling. In fact, falls are extraordinarily common; serious falls are the number-one cause of injury death in those over age 75. (Before age 75, that honor belongs to motor vehicle accidents.) Taking steps to avoid falls, especially in the home, is important for all of us, but especially for older adults. You can get some excellent information on how to fall-proof yourself and your home from:

National Safety Council
1121 Spring Lake Drive
Itasca, IL 60143-3201
(800) 621-7619
www.nsc.org

Finally, workplace injuries contribute to osteoarthritis. We know, for instance, that workers involved in lifting and carrying often have osteoarthritis of the lower back and knees. People who sit at a desk and computer all day frequently get OA of the neck (mainly from bad posture and positioning). People who work with their hands a lot—gardeners and construction workers, for example—commonly get osteoarthritis of the neck, back, and upper extremities, especially their hands. Fortunately, the percentage of workers injured on the job has been declining steadily over the past several years, mainly because of education and improved standards and guidelines for working conditions. I hope this trend continues as employers realize they can lower the cost of business by keeping their employees healthy.

Levels of Osteoarthritis Prevention

Most of my patients ask me, "Dr. Theo, how can I prevent arthritis?" The answer to this question isn't clear-cut, because there are actually several different types of prevention. When we discuss the issue of prevention for arthritis it's important to clear up the subcategories of prevention, because the interventions at each level are quite different.

Arthritis prevention falls into three major types: *primary, secondary* and *tertiary*.

Primary prevention is defined as activities that lessen the chances of an individual or population, without known risk factors, for developing osteoarthritis *before* they have the disease.

Examples of primary prevention activities for osteoarthritis would include:

- Preventing joint injury through strengthening, balance, and agility drills and good coaching for proper technique in sports and daily activities.
- General injury prevention techniques, such as improving driving skills by taking a course and wearing seat belts, and reducing the risk of falls by making changes in the home. In sports, using the proper equipment in the correct way is an important part of primary prevention.
- Avoiding obesity or diabetes by maintaining a healthy body weight.
- Switching from high-risk sports and activities to those with less risk. Biking instead of running, or running on a softer surface instead of cement or asphalt, are good examples.

- Changing the workplace environment to limit acute or chronic mechanical overload of workers' joints.
- Consider using glucosamine/chondroitin and ASU supplements preventively, to help heal minor joint damage before it becomes osteoarthritis. (I'll discuss this in detail under Step 8.)

Secondary prevention of osteoarthritis involves early detection and prompt treatment of this disease as well as conditions known to lead to the development of osteoarthritis. Examples here include:

- Losing weight if you're overweight.
- Detaecting and correcting metabolic diseases such as hyper-parathyroidism, gout, iron overload (hemochromatosis), and dia-betes—diseases that are closely linked to osteoarthritis.
- Avoiding running or other high-impact activities after surgical removal of the meniscus cartilage in the knee.
- Correcting low levels of vitamins C and D.
- Using glucosamine/chondroitin and ASU preventively, especially in the presence of other risk factors.

Tertiary prevention of osteoarthritis can really be considered treat-ment for the diseased joints, limitation of the disability, and rehabilita-tion of disease so the sufferer can attempt to lead as normal a life as possible. Some might even consider joint replacement as a tertiary preventive measure, since replacing a severely damaged joint may help an individual lessen the mechanical forces on other joints and help keep them from developing arthritis. We now know that even people with the most severe cases of osteoarthritis and even those who have already had joint replacement are great candidates to benefit from glucosamine/chondroitin and ASU.

Odd as it sounds, even people with artificial joints can benefit from taking the supplements. Of course, the supplements can't help a joint that isn't there any more, but there is some good evidence to suggest that the supplements may be able to help keep a replaced joint from becoming loose—a common cause of failure in hip and knee replace-ments. Even though the artificial joint is not alive, the interface between the artificial material and the living bone is a dynamic environment. The living bone releases various natural chemicals that can make the implant fail, to the point where the patient may need to undergo another surgery. Basic science studies show that the supplements inhibit the production or effect of these chemicals.[1]

Overlap in Osteoarthritis Prevention Strategies

Despite the clear differences between primary, secondary, and tertiary prevention of osteoarthritis, there is some overlap among prevention strategies. You may be pleased to know that many of the lifestyle changes you can easily implement can affect all levels of prevention. Exercise and weight loss, for instance, exhibit characteristics in all three preventive categories. Joint strengthening, improvements in bio-mechanics, and training with sports-specific drills prior to competition are excellent methods for both primary and secondary osteoarthritis prevention. No primary prevention trials have been performed yet for glucosamine/chondroitin and ASU, but based on the current evidence, glucosamine/chondroitin and ASU can be classified in both the secondary and tertiary preventive categories.

STEP 2 *Ensure Proper Recovery if You Are Injured*

If you do suffer an injury while exercising or participating in sports, make sure that you are completely recovered and rehabilitated *before* resuming your activity. Many active exercisers and athletes are inclined to downplay even serious injuries. How many times have we seen injured basketball or football players playing on tightly bandaged legs? Or a gymnast hurtling over the vaulting horse despite an ankle injury? Stressing an already injured joint can lead to long-term damage that is difficult or impossible to repair. That might be excusable at the Olympics, but why should the rest of us risk greater damage?

If you're injured, see your doctor as quickly as possible. Get specific instructions as to how to care for your injury, and how long you should rest before starting up again. Your doctor may recommend that you take up a different activity to prevent future irreversible damage.

Meanwhile, there are some simple steps you can follow for immediate treatment of sprains or strains that you can still walk on or move with. Try the "RICER" approach:

- **R**est the injured body part. Allowing damaged tissues to heal is critical. If you don't, you increase the risk of causing further damage by reinjuring the tissue.
- **I**ce the injured area as soon as you can. This helps to reduce inflammation and swelling, both of which can slow down the healing process. Put a sock or thin towel between the injured area and the ice and apply the ice for 20 minutes three times a day for a few days.
- **C**ompress the injured area with an elastic (Ace®) bandage or other restrictive device to prevent swelling, but be careful not to wrap it so tightly that it restricts blood flow. (You should be able to easily slip a finger underneath the bandage.) If your skin starts to discolor, or if the area below the bandage starts to swell, the bandage is too tight.
- **E**levate the injured body part to help prevent swelling. This also forces you to rest the injured area. If you are lying down, elevate the injured area so that it is higher than your heart.
- **R**ehabilitate. Once the pain and inflammation are under control, give your body enough time to rest and recover and then start working on rehabilitating the injured area and regaining flexibility and strength. It's better to wait a little longer and rebuild your strength and flexibility before putting on your sweats and "getting out there" again. Once you're over the acute injury, the retraining of the muscles, tendons, and nerves is a crucial step. The greatest risk factor for sustaining an injury is a past history of injury to the same area. For instance, if you've ever sprained an ankle, you're nine times more likely to reinjure that same ankle compared to someone who has never suffered a sprain.

Beware! If you are experiencing severe or unusual pain after an injury, if you hear or feel something "pop," if a joint or limb appears deformed or misshapen, or if anything else seems amiss, see your doctor or go to an emergency room right away.

I hope that someday the treatment of an acute joint injury will be handled as a true emergency, much as we now treat a heart attack or stroke. In the case of a heart attack or stroke, time is of the essence for treatment to restore the blood supply and minimize damage to healthy tissue. Since we know the trigger for normal cartilage cells to turn into "osteoarthritis cells" is a rapid event, it makes sense to try and intervene immediately after an injury. By eliminating the chemical and physical triggers that convert normal, quiet cartilage cells into hypertrophied and hyperactive cells, we may be able to prevent the onset of osteoarthritis right from the start.

As we learn more and more about the process of how osteoarthritis starts, I would not be surprised if several strategies appear to target the disease at its earliest onset. In the future, this will become as commonplace as cleaning a wound after a laceration to prevent infection.

STEP 3 *Eat a Healthful Diet*

We've already looked in detail at the diet that gives the body the nutritional tools it needs to build and maintain healthy joints. This same healthful approach can be used to prevent joint problems from occurring in the first place. Reread chapter 9, and remember to balance your diet by eating the indicated amount of portions from each area.

Limit your intake of animal and trans fats. Not only do these fats add calories to your diet and pounds to your waistline, increasing your chances of heart disease and cancer, but also the fatty acids they contain may actually aggravate swelling and inflammation. If you're an active person who sometimes gets a sprain or a strain, be especially aware of foods that might worsen the inflammation and encourage free radicals to further damage your joints.

Eat foods rich in antioxidants to counteract free radicals, those highly unstable molecules that can cause major damage to body tissues if left unchecked. The antioxidants can also help to minimize tissue damage if you suffer a sprain or strain. Vitamins A, C, and E, plus the mineral selenium, are some of the many antioxidants found in most vegetables and fruits. (Free radicals have also been linked to cancer, heart disease, aging, and degenerative joint disease, so including antioxidants in your diet is an excellent all-around preventive measure.)

Eat foods high in bioflavonoids to help keep the collagen (an important part of the cartilage matrix) strong and resistant to inflammation. Bioflavonoids also prevent free radical damage and help to heal damaged tissue following injury. Fortunately, the bioflavonoids are ubiquitous—they're found in virtually all plant foods, including fresh vegetables, green tea, berries, onions, citrus fruits, and fruits that contain a pit (such as cherries and plums).

STEP 4 *Maintain a Healthy Body Weight*

The connection between being overweight and having arthritis of the knee or hip has been shown in study after study. Let's look at just a few of the most important recent studies.

The classic study showing the link between excess body weight and knee arthritis comes from the long-running Framingham Study, which since 1948 has been tracking the long-term health of some 1,400 people living in that Massachusetts town. In the 1980s, the researchers looked at the incidence of knee arthritis in the group. What they found was that roughly a third of the people—468 in all—had knee arthritis. Among the men, the heaviest men had about 1.5 times the risk of knee arthritis as the lightest men. Among the women, the difference was marked. The heaviest women had over twice the risk of knee arthritis as the lightest.[2] In the 1990s, researchers looked again at the incidence of knee osteoarthritis among the Framingham participants. By now, these people were in their seventies. The researchers compared knee X rays of the participants taken in the early 1980s to new X rays taken eight to ten years later. Of the 598 participants who didn't have knee arthritis in the 1980s, 93 had developed it by the early 1990s. Who got arthritis? Smokers, people who were physically active, and most commonly, women who were overweight. Every ten pounds of extra weight increased the risk of arthritis by 1.4 times.[3]

A study in Sweden in the early 1990s came up with similar results. Of nearly 550 older adults whose knee arthritis had gotten so bad they needed joint replacement surgery, the biggest risk factor was being an overweight woman. Women who were overweight at age 40 had over nine times the risk of serious knee arthritis later in life as women of normal weight.[4]

More recently, two studies have really demonstrated the connection between weight and arthritis. One study in England compared 525 men and women aged over 45 with serious knee arthritis requiring surgery to a matching group that didn't have arthritis. The risk of arthritis went up right along with body weight, to a high of more than 13 times greater in the people who were very heavy. The researchers concluded that if all overweight or obese people lost at least 15 pounds, some 24 percent of knee operations for arthritis could be avoided.[5] The second study looked at the risk factors for patients needing total hip replacement surgery among more than 50,000 people in Sweden. Here too body weight was a significant risk factor, even more so than intensive physical activity at work. Among the heaviest men, the risk of severe hip arthritis was twice that of the lightest men; among the heaviest women, the risk was 3.4 times that of the lightest women.[6]

The good news is that researchers at the Boston University Arthritis Center who have studied the weight/osteoarthritis connection have concluded that weight loss can help prevent the disease. They found that women who lost an average of eleven pounds over the ten-year study period were only about *half* as likely to develop osteoarthritis as those who weighed the same as or more than they did at the beginning of the study.[7]

It's clear that staying slim is a vital step in holding osteoarthritis at bay. Women are particularly susceptible to developing osteoarthritis when they are overweight. But the message is clear for both women and men of all ages: If you are carrying around too many pounds, get rid of them and you'll decrease your risk of osteoarthritis significantly. If you're already slim, stay that way.

STEP 5 *Exercise Regularly*

Proper exercise does to osteoarthritis what a daily apple does to the doctor: It keeps it away. Your preventive exercise program should be built on exercises that allow your joints to move painlessly through their natural rotation. For example, walking, rowing, swimming, cross-country skiing, and cycling help the knee and hip joints by keeping the joints moving and stimulating cartilage nourishment. (Check back to chapter 8 for more on the importance of exercise.) Before becoming a marathon runner, rower, or cyclist, however, get yourself in good shape by gradually increasing your activities. And if you are overweight, your best bet is to begin with lower impact activities such as biking, water jogging, or brisk walking until you get closer to your ideal weight.

Remember that stretching and muscle conditioning are as important as aerobic conditioning. Stretching improves body awareness and makes your movements more graceful even as it reduces the odds of certain kinds of injuries. Yoga is an excellent stretching exercise, but you also need to stretch before and after any other form of exercise.

Strong muscles also play an important role in preventing osteoarthritis by supporting the joint area and absorbing shock. The muscles transfer weight away from the joint, thereby reducing the stress on the cartilage that comes with impact. Any sort of regular exercise helps build strong muscles, but you can improve on the process by doing light resistance training (also called weight training). You don't need to work out like a bodybuilder to get the benefits of resistance training. Half an hour of working with light to moderate weights just a couple of times a week can make big difference in your muscle strength, which in turn can take a lot of stress off your joints. You can easily work out at home using dumbbells and ankle weights or a home weight-training machine, but I strongly suggest that you get started by working with a professional trainer at a fitness center. You'll get much better results, much more quickly and safely. It's important to select the exercises and stretches that are best for you and to learn how to do them correctly.

When choosing a type of anti-osteoarthritis exercise, select something you enjoy. There's much more to exercise than panting and sweating. It can and should be fun!

STEP 6 *Optimize Your Biomechanics to Counteract Stress on Your Joints*

The same biomechanical techniques that help treat osteoarthritis can be used to prevent the disease. Many people unknowingly walk, jump, swing a tennis racket or golf club, or otherwise move in ways that place unnatural stress on their joints. A biomechanical evaluation can detect and set you on the road to correcting these movement "glitches" before they cause serious trouble.

STEP 7 *Consider Preventive Use of Glucosamine/Chondroitin and ASU*

If you have a higher-than-average risk of developing osteoarthritis, but are not yet suffering symptoms, you may help head off trouble by using glucosamine/chondroitin and ASU on a preventive basis. Since to our knowledge, clinical studies have found no significant long-term side effects, the potential risks from taking these supplements is lower than the risks of swallowing a daily aspirin.

How do you know if your risk is higher than average? It is if you fit into any of the categories listed below:

- *You have a genetic predisposition.* Certain forms of osteoarthritis appear to be inherited. The most common type is *primary generalized osteoarthritis,* in which three or more joints are affected for no known reason. Heberden's nodes and Bouchard's nodes are common in those with a genetic predisposition. A second type of inherited osteoarthritis is associated with familial *chondrocalci-nosis,* a disease in which calcium crystals are deposited in carti-lage. Then there's *Stickler Syndrome,* also known as hereditary arthroophthalmopathy, which occurs in about 1 out of every 10,000 people and is characterized by vision problems (usually shortsightedness) and premature degenerative joint disease.

- *You're overweight or obese.* As discussed above, being overweight or obese is a risk for getting osteoarthritis, especially for women, and losing weight can reduce the risk.

- *You have suffered a major trauma or sports injury to a joint.* Injury makes arthritis much more likely.

- *You've had surgery on your joint or some of your cartilage has been torn or removed in the past.* This places you at extremely high risk for osteoarthritis.

- *You engage in repetitive impact-loading activities.* Ballet dancers, pneumatic drill operators, baseball pitchers, and others who engage in certain repetitive motions are at high risk, especially if they use their joints in unintended ways.

- *You have had injuries in the past and you continued to participate in sports activities that have a high risk of injury.* Sports that involve quick turns, running, jumping, and cutting, and especially those that involve collisions, place participants at high risk for future joint injuries. Remember, if you've had an injury you're nine times more likely to reinjure the same area than someone who has not had an injury to the area.

- *You have misaligned bones.* Bone misalignment can lead to unusual stress on the joint and osteoarthritis. This is actually very common in the hips and knees and can lead to early arthritis with no other apparent cause. A sports medicine physician or orthope-dic doctor can help you determine if you have areas of misalign-ment and help find ways (osteopathic manipulation, soft tissue work, or shoe orthotics, for instance) to correct the problem.

- *You have or have had any one of the metabolic diseases that are known to be associated with osteoarthritis.* These include thyroid and parathy-roid disorders, gout, iron overload, and diabetes, to name a few.

If you belong to any of the risk groups, you may want to consider preventive glucosamine/chondroitin and ASU therapy.

Since the use of glucosamine/chondroitin/ASU in a totally healthy person without risk factors for osteoarthritis has not been studied, I have not encouraged use of these supplements as a *primary* preventive agent. This may soon change, however, as new research in this area becomes available.

In studies comparing animals that were given the supplements to those that weren't, the supplements have had a somewhat protective effect on the type of cartilage damage that leads to osteoarthritis. In other words, having the supplements in their system before injury helped limit the severity of the cartilage damage after injury. Researchers think the effect would be very similar in humans, but for obvious ethical reasons there's no way to duplicate the animal studies. If we had a good marker of the disease for humans, such as something in the joint fluid that determines the level of severity of injury to the cartilage, then perhaps a clinical study could be performed. Unfortunately, there is no accepted consensus on any type of marker for detecting osteoarthritis in the earliest stages, 10 or 20 years before pain and disability set in. The gold standard method had been the use of serial X rays to measure the width of the joint space. MRI scans or perhaps high-definition ultrasounds of the joint cartilage will probably become the new standard at some point in the future, but so far these are not yet sensitive enough to track subtle joint damage over time.

The other reason to consider using joint-health supplements as a primary preventive agent is related to the way we perceive injury. Serious athletes, for example, are often unaware that they have minor injuries that can show up as damage on an MRI scan or by direct visualization with arthroscopic surgery. The injuries are there, even though the athlete doesn't have any significant pain or loss of function. This was exemplified in a study that looked at the incidence of abnormal knees, as determined by MRI scans, in basketball players who said they didn't have any knee problems. Over 60 percent of those players without symptoms had abnormalities on their scans, indicating some cartilage damage.[8] A similar type of study has been done on the general population of nonathletes. About 60 percent of those who do not report any back problems have significant abnormalities on MRI scans of their lower back.[9] Some of these people will go on to develop back problems later on in life, but many won't, even though they have spinal abnormalities.[10] What these studies tell us is that although an injury may seem insignificant because it doesn't hurt or swell up, even unnoticed injuries can lead to cartilage damage over time. Perhaps this helps explain why the majority of people age 65 and older have osteoarthritis, whether they have symptoms of pain or not.

Ever since the supplements were introduced in the original edition of *The Arthritis Cure,* most professional athletes have been using them, even if they don't currently have significant or debilitating problems with their joints. Some orthopedic doctors, myself included, believe that this is one of the major reasons professional athletes have been able to play competitively in their sports much longer in recent years.

You don't have to be a professional athlete to want a life that is healthy, active, and pain-free. Glucosamine/chondroitin and ASU can help you attain that.

STEP 8 *Use Joint-Supporting Dietary Supplements*

As discussed in the chapter on healthy eating, it's always best to get your vitamins and minerals from a well-balanced diet rich in fresh fruits and vegetables. In addition to eating well, however, supplements of vitamins A, C, and E and the trace minerals selenium, manganese, and boron are helpful for keeping your joints healthy. Calcium supplements are also helpful for overall bone health. Fish oil and GLA capsules are helpful for reducing inflammation in the joint. Most major medical organizations, including the conservative American Medical Association, have recommended a daily multivitamin for all adults.

Summing Up

The eight-step arthritis prevention program is simple, inexpensive, and easy to follow. All you have to do is decide to do it, and you're already on your way to reducing your risk of osteoarthritis while improving your overall health. Again, be sure to discuss this program with your doctor before starting.

12

RHEUMATIC DISEASE REVIEW

The most common forms of arthritis.

Other diseases that affect the joints.

I t's easy to confuse osteoarthritis and rheumatoid arthritis, two very different rheumatologic diseases with similar names. And it gets even more confusing when you learn that there are more than 100 *different types* of rheumatic diseases, many causing different forms of arthritis. Depending upon the type of arthritis, the associated inflammation may flare up in one joint or many, may limit itself to the joint only, or might spread to the muscles, tendons, ligaments, internal organs, and even the skin. Different types of arthritis have different causes, courses, and cures.

Naturally, your arthritis cannot be effectively treated until the type has been diagnosed. Your doctor will make the diagnosis, which may very well be one of the common forms listed here.

BURSITIS AND TENDONITIS

Many an unhappy weekend athlete is familiar with bursitis and tendonitis: pain and tenderness in the shoulders, elbows, knees, or pelvis that radiates into the nearby limbs and is sometimes accompanied by warmth in the affected areas. Bursitis and tendonitis are the most common forms of soft tissue rheumatic syndromes. They're usually caused by sudden overuse of a joint. It's the areas around the joints of the shoulders, elbows, wrists, fingers, hips, back, knees, ankles, and feet that often pay the price for the overenthusiastic use. Once present, the symptoms can go on for months or years if not treated properly.

Bursa means purse, and the small fluid-filled sacs (bursae) that cushion various parts of the joints do look something like little purses. There are dozens of them in the body; each knee has eight or more. The bursae, which act as cushions (usually between soft tissue and a bony prominence), may become inflamed if a joint is subjected to abnormal pressure. This is most often the result of overuse, a chronic condition, or a trauma such as a fall on the knee or elbow. The bursae can fill with more fluid than usual, triggering pain. Common forms of bursitis are "housemaid's knee" and "student's elbow," which are both caused by leaning too long or too heavily on a joint.

Tendonitis is often grouped with bursitis, but it's actually a very different problem. Tendonitis is characterized by the inflammation or irritation of a tendon, the tough, fibrous, many-layered band of tissue that ties muscles to bones. We normally think that bones only move when muscles contract, but remember that the tendon is "between" the muscle and the bone, allowing the two to work together. Contracting a muscle to move a bone means that the tendons automatically move as well. Forcing swollen tendons to move, however, can be quite painful. Tendonitis is a risk factor for tendon rupture, especially when engaging in ballistic activities (fast takeoffs or jumping).

Tendonitis usually strikes suddenly. It's usually restricted to one area, and can linger for days or weeks before disappearing. Many of us will have tendonitis from overusing or injuring a joint at one time or another in our lives, but fortunately, damage or disability from this condition is rare. It may strike the outside of the elbow as "tennis elbow," the inside of the elbow as "golfer's elbow," the tendons that move the fingers as "trigger finger," the bottom of the pelvis as "weaver's bottom," the finger joints as "video game finger," or the wrist and base of the thumb as de Quervain's disease. Bursitis and tendonitis usually occur after age 30. It's usually the result of wear and tear on tendons, or of abnormal stress on joints or tendons, overambitious workouts by weekend warriors, or a sudden strain, such as lifting a heavy package. Bursitis and tendonitis are usually not chronic conditions, and permanent damage is rare. (Recurring Achilles tendonitis can a sign of ankylosing spondylitis, however, so see your doctor.)

Tendonosis, a variant of tendonitis, is often a chronic condition. Tendonosis refers to a diseased tendon, which is often degenerating on the inside for a variety of possible reasons. This condition is usually not associated with inflammation, which is why the suffix "itis," meaning inflammation, isn't used and the suffix "osis," meaning condition, is attached to the word tendon. Tendonosis is usually diagnosed by either an ultrasound examination or by an MRI scan. Tendonosis can be a very difficult condition to treat since it does not respond to typical anti-inflammatories, stretching, or rest. In some cases, surgeons must intervene and remove the diseased tissue from within the tendon.

A revolutionary new treatment for tendonosis was developed by accident. A man developed chronic Achilles tendon problems (the tendon that runs from your calf muscle down into your heel). Because he lived in a country with socialized medical care, he knew he couldn't have surgery on the tendon until the problem was so severe that the tendon ruptured. He vigorously tried to overload the tendon by doing calf-raising exercises with extremely heavy weights, thinking that this would rupture the tendon and he could then have surgery. Much to his surprise, he found that his tendon problems improved, despite the incredible pain he felt while performing the exercises. Other people tried the same technique, all getting the same results even on other tendons. There is now a great deal of support for purposefully overloading the tendon in order to stimulate its healing. Of course, this should never be tried on your own—if you're having tendon problems, see your doctor and get a specific recommendation.

Treatment of bursitis and tendonitis occurs in phases. Phase I is to remove the aggravating factor(s), use ice and gentle massage on the painful joint, take NSAIDs as appropriate, and do some gentle stretching and range-of-motion exercises. If that doesn't help, Phase II adds physical therapy such as ultrasound or electric stimulation, plus supervised strengthening exercises and moving of the surrounding structures. (Phonophoresis, which involves applying a hydrocortisone cream to the skin and using ultrasound to help the medicine penetrate to the affected area can help relieve pain and inflammation in the tendon. Iontophoresis is similar, but uses an electric current instead of ultrasound.) Phase III brings into play injections of NSAIDs or a cortisonelike drug. Phase IV is surgery, which is rarely needed and is used only if the first three phases do not help after several months.

I often see people who come to me for consultation to treat chronic tennis elbow symptoms. Treatment for tennis elbow starts with rest—no more tennis for a while—and icing the joint three or four times a day for 10 to 15 minutes at a time. At least as important for treatment and preventing future problems is altering the way you use your arms to lift. Since tennis elbow is usually caused by tendonitis or inflammation of the muscles involved in extending the wrist, lifting objects with the palms facing toward the ceiling and not gripping too tightly are the most important ways to rest this inflamed tissue. This can mean a significant alteration in daily activities, such as lifting up a bag or briefcase or even lifting clothes off a hanger. If the sufferer continues to have problems even lifting small items in daily life, then it's very difficult to overcome this condition. Each time you feel pain while lifting something, it's because small microscopic tears are occurring in the newly formed scar tissue the body lays down in an attempt to heal the area. This delays healing further and explains why some people can suffer for months. In addition to changes in how you lift, stretching the muscles in the forearm is critical. The best stretch involves keeping your elbow straight on the affected arm and using your other hand to grab the affected arm's fingers just above the knuckles. Pull steadily on the fingers so that the palm of the affected arm is pulled toward the forearm.

Muscle toning exercises can begin two to three week after the acute pain has subsided. Muscle toning begins with the grip strength and slowly works up to the wrist and then the forearm. A physical therapist or doctor can advise you on the best exercises to do. When doing strengthening exercises, avoid any that cause sharp pain, as this may indicate too much stress on the tendon. A healthy elbow comes about through developing a healthy grip, wrist, forearm, and biceps. Take care to avoid activities that stress any one part of the arm over the others.

GOUT

When someone mentions gout, we usually think of the huge-bellied, gluttonous King Henry VIII swilling port wine and chewing on a leg of mutton, his bandaged foot resting on a stool. Gout was once called the "rich man's disease" because it was associated with being overweight, overeating (especially meat), and overindulging in drink. Today we know that gout is a metabolic disorder, but a poor diet can make the condition worse.

In gout, uric acid, a waste product in the urea (urine) cycle, is either overproduced, underexcreted, or both. When a person has too much uric acid in his or her system, some of it forms uric acid crystals. These crystals (think of them as sharp pieces of glass inside your body) can be deposited into the joint space, rather than being cleared by the kidneys. These "glass shards" often find their way to the "bunion joint" of the big toe, although gout is also found in the other joints of the feet, as well as those of the fingers, wrists, elbows, knees, and ankles. The afflicted joint suddenly becomes hot, painfully swollen, and stiff; fever and chills sometimes follow. The skin of the affected area can appear shiny red or purple. The pain from an acute attack of gout can be excruciating. In some cases, the joint is so tender that even the light brush of a bed sheet can cause howls of pain.

Gout affects about two million Americans, most of them male (80 percent). Risk factors for getting the disease include a family history of gout, drinking alcohol, high blood pressure, taking certain medications, being overweight, or gaining weight unchecked. Aside from the severe pain of a gout attack, the disease can be hazardous to your long-term health. The uric acid crystals may eventually be deposited in soft tissue, cartilage, joints, tendons, or elsewhere, forming painful lumps, and the crystals can also damage the kidneys. The good news is that gout can often be completely controlled with proper treatment, which usually includes the use of nonsteroidal anti-inflammatory drugs (NSAIDs) for pain and inflammation, abstinence from alcohol, dietary restrictions (avoiding foods such as organ meats), and possibly medications to reduce the amount of uric acid production or increase its excretion in the urine.

It is very important to treat gout and prevent gouty attacks because recurrent attacks can lead to joint destruction, deformities, and arthritis in the affected joint. Gout is a common secondary risk factor for osteoarthritis. Treating the gout, and preventing uric acid crystals from getting into the joint, are the most important ways to prevent secondary osteoarthritis.

PSEUDOGOUT

The name makes it sound as if it's a fake, but the pain and other symptoms of pseudogout are real. Often striking the knee joint, then the wrists and ankles, pseudogout attacks suddenly, causing pain and swelling in the joint and possibly destroying cartilage. An attack may go on for days or even weeks, with the acute phase lasting 12 to 36 hours. Sometimes the pain may flare up in several joints at a time, though when that happens pseudogout is usually less severe and more chronic. Sometimes the pain increases after activity; sometimes it doesn't. These symptoms often disappear without treatment.

Also known as calcium pyrophosphate crystal deposition disease, pseudogout is a form of inflammatory arthritis. As is the case with gout, the pain is caused by crystals deposited in the joint spaces, but in pseudogout the crystals are formed from calcium pyrophosphate rather than uric acid. The calcium crystals can also be deposited into the cartilage, causing a condition called chondrocalcinosis (Latin for "calcium in the cartilage").

Pseudogout is uncommon before the age of 65 and it seems to affect men and women equally. The disease can be brought on by surgery, trauma, or stress (because stress causes excessive parathyroid hormone production, which affects the calcium balance in your body). Unlike gout, it's not caused or affected by diet. Even though the crystals contain calcium, drinking milk or eating high-calcium foods doesn't seem to make a difference.

Treatment includes joint aspiration to remove the fluid containing the crystals and NSAIDs to manage pain and inflammation. Exercise helps to build muscle strength and restore full motion of the joints after an acute attack. In rare instances, surgery may be used to replace a joint that has been badly damaged, is extremely painful, or is unstable.

Perhaps the most dramatic responses to glucosamine and chondroitin I have ever seen occurred in people suffering from pseudogout. Some cases were patients who had little response to NSAIDs or even cortisone injections and who were contemplating radical surgeries to scrape down the cartilage and calcium deposits. After a few weeks on the supplements, their recovery was dramatic. Some were completely cured of their pain and swelling, even years later, and even after they took up running again. Glucosamine has an "antireactive" effect that helps keep the calcium crystals from irritating the cartilage. This is why I believe that the research on the supplements, which generally just includes people with *primary* osteoarthritis, underestimates the real-world value of treating people with joint pain from other types of arthritis.

INFECTIOUS ARTHRITIS

Can arthritis be brought about by germs? Absolutely. Many forms of bacteria, viruses, and fungi can cause infectious arthritis, which is frequently characterized by loss of joint function, fever, and inflammation of one or more joints, and (occasionally) chills. The knee joint is most commonly involved (50 percent of the cases), followed by the hip, shoulder, wrist, and ankle. Infectious arthritis can generally be cured if caught early enough. In practice, any bacterium, virus, or fungus that produces disease can prompt this infectious form of arthritis, and there are many ways that the infecting agent can enter the body: trauma, surgery, inserting a needle into a joint, abscess or bone infection near the joint, animal bites, insect bites (see the discussion of Lyme disease that follows), and even thorns. Chronic alcoholics and drug abusers are at high risk for infectious arthritis, as are those suffering from diabetes, sickle-cell anemia, kidney disease, and certain forms of cancer. A less obvious cause of joint infection is bacteria that travels through the bloodstream from a distant site in the body and settles in a joint. Infections almost anywhere in the body can move to the joints, including infections that begin in the lungs, urinary tract, and skin. Remember that any medical procedure involving a joint can lead to infection and infectious arthritis. Many joint infections are complications of surgery on the joints; very rarely does an injection into the joint space actually lead to an infection.

The body responds to the infection by mobilizing the immune system and engaging in a fierce battle with the infectious agent. The joint becomes the battleground. Like all battlegrounds, the joint suffers, becoming inflamed and painful as the body releases enzymes that inadvertently degrade the cartilage as they seek to destroy the invaders.

The goal in treating infectious arthritis is first to eliminate the infection, then handle the arthritis itself. Treatment depends upon what caused it in the first place: antibiotics are prescribed for bacterial causes, while NSAIDs are the medicine of choice for viral causes. If the cause is a bacterial infection, infected joints should be drained in order to limit destruction to the joint due to the active infection and inflammation. Physical therapy may then be used to build up muscle strength and relieve joint stiffness.

LYME DISEASE

A bacterial illness caused by a spirochete, Lyme disease is spread by bites from infected deer ticks. The illness gets its name from Old Lyme, Connecticut, where the first cases were recognized in 1975. Today it is the most common tick-transmitted disease in the United States. It's most common in the northeastern region, but cases have been reported in every state and also in other countries.

Lyme disease usually, though not always, starts with a characteristic "bull's-eye" rash at the site of the tick bite. This is followed by flu-like symptoms, including fever, muscle and joint pain, and headaches. When Lyme disease patients are treated promptly with antibiotics, the illness usually goes away with no lasting effects. Unfortunately, because the bull's-eye rash isn't always present and because the other symptoms can sometimes be quite mild, some patients don't know they have the disease and go untreated. These people can end up with late-stage nerve and heart problems—and also with arthritis, usually in the knees. In fact, the first cases of Lyme disease were initially diagnosed as rheumatoid arthritis because the patients all suddenly had swollen, painful knee joints. It was only when doctors realized that a cluster of rheumatoid arthritis cases in one place at one time was unlikely that they realized there was an infection involved.

As with other forms of infectious arthritis, treatment for late-stage Lyme disease usually involves antibiotics to treat the infection and NSAIDs and possibly surgery to treat the affected joints.

JUVENILE ARTHRITIS

A temperature that swings up and down on a daily basis, chills, possibly a body rash, plus pain or swelling in the toes, knees, ankles, elbows, or shoulders are the hallmarks of juvenile arthritis.

Juvenile arthritis is a general term for the various kinds of arthritis that can strike children under the age of 16. The most common form that children in the United States suffer from is juvenile rheumatoid arthritis (JRA). JRA appears in three distinct forms: *systemic, polyarticular, and pauciarticular*, with the common characteristics of joint inflammation (stiffness, swelling, pain, warmth, and redness).

In *systemic JRA* (also known as Still's disease), there is usually a fever of 103° or more which disappears in a few hours, only to reappear the next day. This high temperature may be accompanied by shaking, swollen lymph nodes, and a rash with a peculiar salmon-pink color that comes and goes. These signs and symptoms may last for weeks or even months. Many joints can be affected; the disease can also affect the blood and the outer lining of the heart or lungs. There may also be stomach pain, severe anemia, and a high white-cell count. Systemic JRA should always be closely monitored by a physician.

Polyarticular JRA appears in several joints (five or often strikes more). Like rheumatoid arthritis (see below), it often strikes symmetrically, affecting the same joint on both sides of the body (such as both knees). In some cases, the patient may also suffer a slight fever and eye inflammation. Girls are more likely to contract the long-term disease, which can extend into adulthood and is thought to be the same as adult rheumatoid arthritis. Another type of polyarticular JRA seems to strike mostly boys. This form is characterized by stiffness in the upper and lower back, arthritis in the large joints, and often develops into ankylosing spondylitis as the child reaches adulthood.

Pauciarticular JRA affects only a few joints, most often the large ones such as the knee, ankle, or elbow. It is not usually symmetrical. Because of the pain, children with arthritis tend to avoid moving their inflamed joints. As a result, the unused joints can become chronically stiff and the surrounding muscles weak. In rare instances, long-term inflammation can damage the joint surfaces, causing deformity. In this type of JRA there is a very high risk of eye inflammation (uveitis) so children with this disease need regular eye exams. This type of eye inflammation can lead to blindness if undetected or untreated.

We don't know what causes JRA. However, it is not contagious and rarely appears in more than one child in a family. The disease is usually treated with aspirin and other NSAIDS. When the disease is unresponsive to these anti-inflammatory medications, powerful immunosuppressive agents such as sulfasalazine, methotrexate, cyclosporin and azothioprin (Imuran®) are used, as well as low doses of corticosteroids. The newly introduced biologic medications, including etanercept (Enbrel®), adalimumab (Humira®), and infliximab (Remicade®) are very effective in treating JRA that is not responsive to traditional medications. These agents can have remarkable results in treating children with JRA by eliminating the joint inflammation and slowing or reversing the disease enough to prevent joint deformities and disability.

Exercise is very important in JRA because it helps to prevent stiffness and maintain muscle strength. Surgery may be necessary to correct severe joint damage.

RHEUMATOID ARTHRITIS (RA)

Rheumatoid arthritis (RA) is an autoimmune disease brought about when the body has, for unknown reasons, turned on itself. In RA, the immune system starts attacking body tissues as if they were foreign invaders. In its mildest form, rheumatoid arthritis is characterized by joint discomfort caused when the joint lining, especially the part that meets the cartilage, becomes inflamed. In its most serious form, RA can cause painfully deformed joints and harm organ systems.

Some experts believe that RA is brought about by a bacterial infection in the joints, but it might also be triggered by a virus in those who are genetically susceptible. People with a family history of RA have a much higher risk of RA. A recent study suggests that the disease's origin may be related to the body's attack on a carbohydrate chain in the joint cartilage, not on proteins, as had been previously been theorized.

Over time, the chronic inflammation of RA makes the joint lining thick and overgrown. This overgrown lining may then start to invade the cartilage, other joint-supporting tissues, and even the bone, causing small erosions in the bone and weakening the entire joint structure. Eventually, the weakened joint becomes more and more painful and less able to perform. Under pressure, it may even become dislocated and deformed.

Usually appearing in the same joint on both sides of the body (both hands, for example), RA hits suddenly. The joints become swollen, tender, and inflamed; there may also be fever, weight loss, and a general feeling of sickness, soreness, stiffness, and aching. The eyes and mouth may dry out if the tear and salivary glands become involved. People with RA generally have stiffness in their joints that lasts for an hour or more when they wake up in the morning. The pain and stiffness are often better after movement.

RA affects more than 2.5 million people in the United States, striking women three times as often as men. Onset is typically between the ages of 20 and 40, although older persons and children are also victims. Joint inflammation is chronic and can be mild to severe, with occasional attacks or "flares." The disease may get progressively worse over time and lead to severe deformities in the joints

The treatment for RA is designed to alleviate pain, reduce inflammation, stop or slow joint damage, and improve overall body functioning. In the past, treatment was started with mostly mild drugs; the more potent (and potentially more hazardous) disease-modifying drugs (or DMARDs) were reserved for the time when the disease started to cause joint destruction. The trend over the past few years, however, has been to start with more aggressive treatment immediately rather than wait for joint destruction to become apparent. Some rheumatoid arthritis sufferers can have rapid progression of the disease. In just a year they can have such severe damage to one or two joints that they require joint replacement surgery. This is why it's critical to get a diagnosis of RA early, have a consultation with a rheumatologist, and start prescription medicine immediately. Aspirin and NSAIDs are used to control pain in RA, but these drugs do not slow the progression of the joint destruction. Immunosuppressive medications such as methotrexate, sulfasalazine, leflunomide (Arava®), hydroxychloroquine, azothioprin (Imuran), and cyclosporin may help slow the joint destruction associated with RA. Three new biologic medicines known as tumor necrosis factor inhibitors have been approved for use in RA: etanercept (Enbrel), infliximab (Remicade) and adilimumab (Humira). Another new medication called anakinra (Kineret®), which works by blocking the activity of a natural inflammatory agent in your body called interleukin-1, is now available. These medications have had a major impact on controlling pain, joint swelling, and joint destruction due to RA. Exercise and therapy can help reduce joint soreness and swelling, alleviate pain, and increase joint mobility. Surgery is an option in the case of severe damage to the hips or knees and sometimes the shoulder when it can make the difference between dependence and independence.

Unfortunately, there have not been any large, controlled studies on the use of glucosamine, chondroitin, or ASU on rheumatoid arthritis sufferers. From a theoretical standpoint, some of the mechanisms of action of these supplements would suggest that they should benefit. The supplements can inhibit the enzymes that break down cartilage as well as the negative effects of IL-1, chemicals that are produced both in osteoarthritis and even more so in rheumatoid arthritis. Furthermore, many people with RA also have osteoarthritis and can benefit from the use of the supplements. Since every case of RA is different, it is important to discuss the use of these supplements with your rheumatologist.

PSORIATIC ARTHRITIS
Psoriatic arthritis is an inherited disease that sometimes occurs in people with the skin condition called psoriasis. The red, scaly patches of psoriasis often appear on the neck, knees, and elbows; the nails may become pitted. People with psoriatic arthritis usually have stiffness in their joints in the morning that lasts at least 30 minutes. Psoriatic arthritis often affects the back. It also often affects the end joints of the fingers or toes, causing them to become so swollen that they're often referred to as "sausage digits." Despite the swelling, affected joints tend to be less tender than with other arthritis conditions, so patients with psoriatic arthritis may develop joint deformity without a significant amount of pain.

Although swollen joints in the extremities are the most common symptom of psoriatic arthritis, the diagnosis can't be made unless the patient also has skin and nail involvement consistent with psoriasis. Sometimes, however, patients with psoriatic arthritis have only nail lesions or such mild skin lesions that they don't even know they have psoriasis.

Psoriatic arthritis usually appears when its victims are between the ages of 20 and 30, although it may occur at any age. It affects men and women equally, and occurs in 5 to 8 percent of those who have psoriasis. Treatment regimens include NSAIDs to reduce the inflammation, exercises to improve joint mobility, and immunosuppressive dugs such as methotrexate or cyclosporin, which can slow the rate of joint destruction. The new biologic medications etanercept and infliximab have been approved for the treatment of psoriatic arthritis and can be very effective at both clearing up the skin lesions and treating the arthritis.

ANKYLOSING SPONDYLITIS

If you wake up in the morning with lower back pain and stiffness, if you've had the low back pain for longer than three months, and if it gets better with exercise but is not improved with rest, you may have ankylosing spondylitis (AS).

Causing fused spinal vertebrae, AS is most commonly seen in young men. It sometimes goes untreated in earlier stages because it can easily be confused with mechanical back pain, the kind you get from lifting a heavy object. With AS, the tendons and ligaments that move the back become inflamed. The vertebrae respond to the problem by producing more bone. The body's response is well intentioned, but making extra bone can cause the vertebrae to grow into each other and fuse together. Eventually, the spine can wind up looking like a bamboo pole. It gets so stiff that the natural inward curvature of the low back and the natural extension of the neck are lost, making AS sufferers appear bent over. They don't really have trouble holding up their heads—their neck vertebrae are fused in that position. If you have ever seen an elderly person walking bent over as though he were looking at his shoes, you have probably witnessed the late stages of AS.

AS inflammation usually begins in the lower back, and always involves the sacroiliac joints (the joints where the lower spine meets the pelvis). In later stages the middle and upper back and neck are afflicted. The disease can spread down into the buttocks and thighs, or up into the chest, where it can make deep breaths difficult. The inflammation may also strike the joints of the shoulder, knees, or ankles. It can also affect the eyes—about 30 percent of patients with AS will develop anterior uveitis (inflammation of the iris) at some point. In fact, in some 20 percent of AS cases, the first signs of arthritis appear in the knees, hips, heels, or eyes.

Young men between 16 and 35 years of age are the favorite targets of AS, which afflicts approximately 1 in 1,000 people under the age of 40. Three times as many males as females are diagnosed with the disease, but this may be because females tend to have much milder symptoms and may never be diagnosed. It also appears in children (mostly boys), who account for roughly 5 percent of the cases. It is rarely seen in African-Americans.

Scientists have found what may prove to be a genetic basis for AS. The disease is found almost exclusively in those who have the HLA-B27 gene, a gene involved in fighting infection. But don't worry if you carry HLA-B27—less than 5 percent of those with the gene eventually develop the disease. It's not enough simply to have the genetic tendency—the gene has to be "switched on" somehow. (If one identical twin develops AS, it appears in the other twin only 60 percent of the time.) Studies currently under way are looking into the possibility that a certain type of infection triggers AS.

Early diagnosis and proper treatment of AS can reduce or prevent deformity. The treatment regimens are designed to reduce pain and prevent deformities, while strengthening the back and neck. Non-steroidal anti-inflammatory drugs (NSAIDs) are used to reduce pain and inflammation but do not prevent progression of the disease. Exercise and posture improvement help to increase strength and flexibility. The new biologic agents infliximab and etanercept show great promise in the treatment of AS. Not only do they help decrease pain and increase flexibility in patients with AS, they can also slow or even stop progression of the disease. In July 2003 etanercept (Enbrel) was approved by the FDA for treatment of AS.

Glucosamine and chondroitin are often used by AS sufferers, but mainly in an effort to decrease their reliance on NSAIDs. Some patients report that the supplements help, but no formal studies on these supplements or ASU have been done yet.

REACTIVE ARTHRITIS

Like ankylosing spondylitis, reactive arthritis can affect the back, peripheral joints, and eyes. Unlike AS, however, reactive arthritis is definitely brought on by an infection. The precipitating infection is usually an enteric infection (one causing diarrhea) or a genital infection such as chlamydia or gonorrhea, but sometimes the infection is asymptomatic and the patient never feels sick or knows he or she had an infection. The arthritis symptoms usually develop one to four weeks after the triggering infection. The pain and swelling occurs most commonly in the lower limbs. The patients usually have morning stiffness lasting at least one hour; they also usually feel tired and sometimes have a fever. They sometimes will also have back pain that is worse after rest and improved with exercise. Most patients with reactive arthritis have only one episode of arthritis and then the symptoms go away completely. Anywhere from 15 to 50 percent of patients will have recurrence of the arthritis at some time, however, and about 20 percent of patients with reactive arthritis develop a chronic arthritis that can affect both the limbs and the back. NSAIDs are usually the initial treatment for reactive arthritis. If the symptoms persist, patients are often started on stronger drugs such as methotrexate or sulfasalazine.

Other Diseases That Affect the Joints

Arthritis is not the only disease that attacks the joints. Other diseases, arising in various parts of the body, may damage the joints as a side effect. The diseases discussed below are not truly forms of arthritis, but they can cause arthritis-like symptoms.

FIBROMYALGIA

Characterized by widespread, sometimes incapacitating pain, fibromyalgia produces stiffness and weakness of the muscular areas of the lower back, hips, thighs, neck, shoulder, chest, or arms, accompanied by muscle spasms ("charley horses") in any of those areas. Patients often tell their doctors: "I hurt all over." The symptoms of fibromyalgia are quite similar to those of chronic fatigue syndrome (CFS), which explains why doctors have had a hard time distinguishing between the two. But in recent years, researchers have discovered that the diagnosis of fibromyalgia is based on pain or tenderness in at least 11 of 18 specific points of the body.

Formerly referred to as fibrositis, because it was thought to be an inflammation of the muscles, fibromyalgia literally means "muscle pain." Recent controlled studies, however, show no evidence of inflamed muscles in patients with fibromyalgia. Researchers now think that fibromyalgia is secondary to abnormal pain perception. In controlled studies, patients with fibromyalgia perceived stimuli as painful at lower levels than did controls. When the brain activity of patients with fibromyalgia was compared to that of controls, people with fibromyalgia had more brain activity in response to the same stimuli. In other words, someone with fibromyalgia is very sensitive to pain. Things that someone without fibromyalgia doesn't perceive as painful are definitely painful to people with fibromyalgia. Why this is so is still a mystery.

Women between the ages of 35 and 60 are the most likely victims of fibromyalgia, with the highest incidence occurring just before menopause. No specific cause has been pinpointed. Fibromyalgia is often misdiagnosed because most of its symptoms are similar to those found in other conditions.

Treatment of fibromyalgia includes alleviating chronic pain and sleep disturbances, as well as dealing with the depression that often accompanies a chronic disease. Water exercises, biofeedback, and relaxation techniques are all helpful. Although aspirin and NSAIDs are usually prescribed to relieve the pain, they don't always do the job. That's why muscle relaxants or local anesthetics are sometimes injected into the painful areas to quickly relax the muscle and alleviate pain. In addition, medications that act on the central nervous system, most notably the prescription drugs amitriptyline (Elavil®) and cyclobenzaprine (Flexeril®), have been shown to help sleep disturbance and improve pain. SSRI antidepressants such as fluoxetine (Prozac®) also seem to help with pain due to fibromyalgia, even if the patient isn't depressed. Fibromyalgia is a very difficult disease, both to have and to treat. The good news is that although the joints may be painful, the disease does not cause deformity or deterioration.

PAGET'S DISEASE

Also known as osteitis deformans, Paget's disease is a bone disorder characterized by bone pain and deformity. In this disease the normal process of bone remodeling (breakdown and build-up) speeds up markedly. New, bulkier, and softer bone is produced, but it's weaker and has a greater tendency to fracture than does normal bone. Paget's disease most often strikes the bones of the pelvis, skin, spine, and the long bones of the leg. The weakened bone structure characteristic of the disease leads to arthritis in the nearby joints. Ringing in the ears and hearing loss may occur if the small bones of the ear have been targeted by the disease. Over time, the rapid bone formation gradually stops. The symptoms may appear and disappear, but any bone alteration or damage that has already occurred is permanent.

Paget's disease doesn't usually have any symptoms at the onset, so the early presence of the disease can only be detected by routine blood tests. When symptoms do arise, they can best be described, as "deep bone pain," a feeling of warmth all over, or headaches if the skull bones are affected. Bones are chronically painful (especially at night); they seem to be getting larger and the skin that covers them feels unusually warm. Bone formation is altered as the disease progresses, causing a weakening, thickening, and deformity of the bones. Movement may be impaired and the bones may fracture easily.

Paget's disease is more common in men than in women, and often surfaces between the ages of 50 and 70. It may run in families. Most of those affected are of northwestern European ancestry, although the disease is occasionally seen in African-Americans. The cause of Paget's disease is unknown. Treatment centers on relieving pain, preventing bone deformity or fracture, and protecting hearing. Alendronate (Fosamax®), a medication used for osteoporosis, is also given to patients with Paget's disease. Surgery may be used to correct both hearing loss and bowed bones.

POLYMYOSITIS AND DERMATOMYOSITIS

Commonly referred to as myositis, these two diseases are characterized by inflammation of the connective tissues. In polymyositis, the inflammation leads to weakening and subsequent breakdown of the muscles; in dermatomyositis, the skin is affected.

Polymyositis produces an inflammation of the muscle (especially in the arms and legs) that leads to the destruction of muscle fiber and makes the muscle waste away. If the shoulder is involved, the patient will have difficulty reaching up to comb his or her hair or to take a dish out of the cupboard. If muscles in the hip area are attacked, it may become difficult for a person to get out of a chair or climb stairs. In its most severe form, polymyositis can weaken muscles in the neck and throat, changing the voice and making it difficult to swallow. If chest muscles are affected, it may become hard to breathe.

In dermatomyositis, the skin is affected and becomes very tender. A reddish patchy rash can appear on the face, knuckles, elbows, knees, ankles, or around the eyes. Sometimes the eyelids will become puffy and have a purplish color. In more advanced cases, rubbing a finger across the affected area can take off several layers of skin.

Other symptoms of polymyositis and dermatomyositis include fever, weight loss, and joint pain. No one knows exactly what causes myositis, although it has many similarities to lupus and rheumatoid arthritis and is probably the result of hypersensitivity or autoimmune problems. Myositis appears gradually over a period of months. It usually strikes people between the ages of 30 and 60, and affects twice as many women as men. Most patients respond well to treatment, although it can be fatal in some, particularly older people who also have cancer.

Myositis is usually treated with corticosteroids. Methotrexate is often used to decrease the amount of prednisone necessary to control the disease. Intravenous immunoglobulin therapy has been beneficial in those patients with myositis who do not respond to steroids. Physical therapy is extremely important to help rebuild the muscle strength that is lost because of the disease.

SCLERODERMA

Scleroderma means "thick skin," so it's no wonder that the disease is characterized by a hardening and thickening of the skin on the hands, arms, and face, as well as ulcers on the fingers, hair loss, and discoloration. It also affects the joints, blood vessels, and internal organs.

Women are affected by scleroderma five times more often than men. The disease's favorite targets are women between the ages of 30 and 60, although it can strike either sex at any age. Like rheumatoid arthritis, scleroderma is believed to be an autoimmune disease triggered by an unknown factor. The trigger may be environmental or chemical (sclerodermalike diseases have been seen in workers who are exposed to silica dust or vinyl chloride, as well as in people taking the cancer drug bleomycin or the amino acid supplement L-tryptophan). Patients receiving bone marrow transplants sometimes develop a condition that closely resembles scleroderma.

The body's tiny blood vessels and capillaries become inflamed when scleroderma strikes, which in turn prompts the body to overproduce collagen, the protein that makes up most of the connective tissues. The excess collagen is deposited in the skin and body organs, where it hardens, causing the skin to thicken and the internal organs to malfunction. Although the joints themselves aren't damaged by scleroderma, they may feel stiff because the skin over them has become hard. Indeed, the fingers may become stiff and clawlike as excess cartilage is deposited, even though the joints themselves are still healthy. The most severe complications of the disease are related to the buildup of collagen in internal organs and the scarring that causes. Scleroderma-induced damage to the esophagus, heart, lungs, kidneys, or intestinal tract can be fatal.

There is no cure for scleroderma, but several medications are used to control the symptoms. These include aspirin and NSAIDs for pain and inflammation, corticosteroids for muscle problems, antacids for heartburn, and medications to control high blood pressure and stimulate circulation. Careful exercise helps to maintain overall fitness and to keep the skin and joints flexible. Protecting the skin from further damage is also an important part of the treatment of scleroderma.

SJÖGREN'S SYNDROME

After rheumatoid arthritis, Sjögren's syndrome, also known as kerato-conjunctivitis sicca, is the most common autoimmune rheumatic disease. It inflames the tear and saliva glands, causing dry eyes and mouth. Itchy, red, irritated eyes and double vision are common symptoms, as well as cracks in the tongue or at the corners of the mouth, difficulty chewing, and swallowing, and a decreased sense of taste. Other problems associated with Sjögren's syndrome include fatigue, dental cavities, joint inflammation, and inflammation of the lungs, kidneys, liver, nerves, thyroid gland, and brain. A mild form of arthritis usually accompanies the condition.

Sjögren's syndrome is often found in conjunction with other autoimmune diseases such as lupus, rheumatoid arthritis, or scleroderma. Although no specific cause has been determined, it is believed that heredity, viral infections, and hormones maybe important factors in the disease. Sjögren's can strike anyone at any time, but 90 percent of those who get it are women, and it is rare among those under the age of 20.

Treatment is designed to relieve discomfort while controlling mouth and eye dryness. Lubricating eye drops, chewing gum, and, room humidifiers may be helpful. Aspirin and NSAIDs are used to reduce joint pain, inflammation, and muscle aches. Exercise can help to keep joints and muscles flexible.

SYSTEMIC LUPUS ERYTHEMATOSUS

Also known as lupus, systemic lupus erthyematosus (SLE) is an autoimmune disease that attacks and inflames connective tissues throughout the body. People with SLE may have a red rash spread across the bridge of their noses and cheeks. Because the rash resembles muzzle markings on wolves, the name of the disease come from *lupus*, the Latin word for wolf.

Affecting nine times as many women as men, lupus usually strikes people between the ages of 18 and 45; it is found in about 1 out of 2,000 people. The disease causes the production of abnormal antibodies, and people who have it almost always have a positive blood test for certain antinuclear antigen antibodies (ANA). The skin, kidneys, nervous system, muscles, lungs, bone marrow, and heart can all be affected, as well as the joints (especially the fingers, wrists, and knees). In addition to the red rash on the face, common symptoms include joint pain, mouth sores, stiffness, fever, muscle ache, weight loss, loss of hair, and exhaustion. Some people are also sensitive to ultraviolet light, with exposure to the sun worsening the rash and even making the disease more active. As the disease progresses, inflammation of the linings of the heart, lungs, and kidneys can cause permanent damage.

As with scleroderma and rheumatoid arthritis, an unknown trigger may set lupus in motion, but only in those who are already genetically susceptible. It occurs more often in African-Americans than it does in whites, and some data suggest that Asian and Hispanic populations also have a higher incidence than do whites. Some lupus patients have also been found to be lacking in a certain enzyme involved in healthy immune responses and thus maybe more likely to fall victim to the disease.

The degree of severity of the disease varies quite a bit from person to person. Some don't even know they have it and require no treatment at all, while for others it is a major illness. The majority of people, however, have moderate symptoms and function quite well.

The treatment of lupus includes aspirin and other NSAIDs for pain and inflammation, an antimalarial drug for active attacks or when an extensive rash is present, ointments or skin creams to treat the rashes (sunscreen and avoiding sun exposure are important to prevent the rash), and corticosteroids in severe cases. Drugs such as azathiopirne (Imuran®), methotrexate, mycophenolate (CellCept®), or cyclosporin may be needed to suppress the immune system. If the kidneys are affected lupus is sometimes treated with a powerful medicine called cycophosamide (Cytoxan®) given in high doses to really suppress the immune system. Exercise, avoiding sun exposure, and resting during the active stages of the disease are also important. There have been no clinical studies looking at the benefits of the supplements glucosamine/chondroitin or ASU for lupus, but as with rheumatoid arthritis there are some theoretical reasons to consider the supplements as an adjunct to prescription drugs.

POLYMYALGIA RHEUMATICA

Polymyalgia rheumatica (PMR) is a condition characterized by stiffness and aching originating in the muscles of the neck, shoulder, and hips, especially in the morning. Patients often complain that they just can't get out of bed in the morning due to their stiffness and extreme fatigue. PMR affects approximately 7 people per 1,000 and rarely occurs before the age of 50. Symptoms are due to inflammation and patients can develop swelling in the feet and hands. People with PMR often have trouble moving their shoulders and hips because of the pain. They are not generally weak but can develop weakness due to muscle atrophy and lack of use.

The cause of the discomfort and stiffness found among patients with PMR is inflammation. The location of the inflammation is disputed; it may be in or near large joints such as the hip and shoulder. Peripheral joints may also be involved and arthritis can occur in the small joints of the hands and feet. When these smaller joints are affected the arthritis is usually mild, may be transient, and resolves promptly upon treatment with anti-inflammatory corticosteroids, such as prednisone. Some patients develop swelling due to increased tissue fluid in the hands, wrists, ankles, or the top of the feet. Pitting edema (when a depression remains in swollen tissue after it is pressed) may occur along with other signs of polymyalgia rheumatica, but it can also be the first sign of the disease. Swelling of the tissues of the wrist may lead to symptoms of carpal tunnel syndrome, which occurs in approximately 10 to 15 percent of patients with PMR.

In addition to the swelling, PMR patients may have a decreased ability to actively move the shoulders, neck, and hips. The shoulders may be tender to touch, but this is usually less prominent than expected, given the severity of the symptoms. Muscle strength is usually normal, though weakness may become a problem if the muscles atrophy from disuse due to pain. People with PMR may also develop a related condition called temporal arteritis (see below). Corticosteroids are the standard treatment for PMR, and are usually effective, but they have their side effects. Physical therapy is also important to gain strength lost from disuse during active disease.

TEMPORAL ARTERITIS

Temporal arteritis (TA) is an inflammatory disease of the large and medium-sized arteries in the body. Its symptoms include pain, aching, and stiffness in the muscles of the upper arms, trunk, legs (particularly in the morning), a headache that usually pounds away in one temple, tenderness, swelling, and redness following the path of the temporal artery on one side of the head, pain in the jaw when chewing, vision loss, mild fever, fatigue, and loss of appetite. TA affects the arteries in the cranial branches of the aortic arch, preventing them from delivering an adequate blood supply to the cranial nerves, which are responsible for our vision and muscles in the face. Because of this, people with temporal arteritis often have vision problems, including transient or permanent loss of vision in one eye. The condition can lead to blindness. Approximately 50 percent of patients with temporal arteritis also have polymyalgia rheumatica, but only about 15 percent of patients with PMR develop temporal arteritis.

Doctors use a variety of medicines to treat TA, including corticosteroids and medicines to suppress the immune system.

SUPPLEMENTS AND RHEUMATIC DISEASES

To date there has been little published research on the use of glucosamine/chondroitin and ASU for rheumatic diseases other than osteoarthritis, although there is increasing interest in them in the scientific community. Many people with these conditions use glucosamine/chondroitin anyway, even though there are no supporting studies. The supplements may be effective. The beneficial mechanisms of action for glucosamine, chondroitin, and ASU overlap with many features of other rheumatic diseases, so there is certainly a theoretical basis for their use. Because the supplements are very safe, using them almost certainly won't hurt and may well help. I follow the latest research in these areas very carefully. Check my Web site at www. drtheo.com for the latest news.

ASU has been used in Europe as a treatment for scleroderma with some success. If you have this condition, discuss the use of ASU with your doctor before you try it. ASU has become available in the United States only recently, so your doctor may not know about it yet.

Proven, disease-modifying treatments are now available for many rheumatic diseases. If you have such a condition, always discuss the use of glucosamine, chondroitin, and ASU with your doctor before trying them. Do not start using the supplements on your own; don't stop taking your prescription medication or change the dose without talking to your doctor. Remember, we don't have enough studies yet to know if the supplements help other rheumatic conditions. Any decision to try them should be made in partnership with your doctor under his or her careful supervision.

References

Chapter 1: Can Osteoarthritis Be Cured?

1. Centers for Disease Control, "Prevalence of Disability and Associated Health Conditions—United States, 1991–1992." *Mortality and Morbidity Weekly Review,* 43(40), 1994, pages 730–731, 737–739.

2. Ibid.

3. Yelin, E. and Callahan, L. F. (National Arthritis Data Work Group), "The Economic Costs and Social and Psychological Impact of Musculoskeletal Condition." *Arthritis and Rheumatism,* 38(10), 1995, pages 1351–1362.

4. Report in American College of Rheumatology 64th Annual Scientific Meeting. *Arthritis and Rheumatism,* 43(9 supplement), 2000, page S220.

5. McKenzie, L. S., Horsburgh, B. A., Ghosh, R., and Taylor, T. K. E., "Osteo-arthrosis: Uncertain Rationale for Anti-inflammatory Drug Therapy." *Lancet,* 1, 1976, pages 908–909.

6. Vidal y Plana, R. R., Bizzardi, D., and Rovati, A. L., "Articular Cartilage Pharmacology: In Vitro Studies on Glucosamine and Nonsteroidal Anti-inflammatory Drugs." *Pharmacological Research Communications,* 10(6), 1978, pages 557–569.

7. Palmoski, J. J., and Brandt, K. D., "Effects of Some Non-steroidal Anti-inflammatory Drugs on Proteoglycan Metabolism and Organization in Canine Articular Cartilage." *Arthritis and Rheumatism,* 23, 1980, pages 1010–1020.

8. Felson, D. T., Zhang, Y., Hannan M. T., "Risk Factors for Incident Radi-ographic Knee Osteoarthritis in the Elderly: The Framingham Study." *Arthritis and Rheumatism,* 40, 1997, pages 728–733.

9. Lanyon, P., Muir, K., Doherty, S., and Doherty, M., "Assessment of a Ge-netic Contribution to Osteoarthritis of the Hip: Sibling Study." *British Medical Journal,* 321, 2000, pages 1179–1183.

10. Griffin, M., et al., "Practical Management of Osteoarthritis." *Archives of Family Medicine,* 4, December 1995, pages 1049–1055.

11. Swedberg, J.A., and Steinbauer, J.R., "Osteoarthritis." *American Family Physician,* 45(2), February 1992, pages 557–568.

12. Tsang, J.K., "Update on Osteoarthritis." *Canadian Family Physician,* 36(614), 1990, pages 539–544.

13. Lawrence, R.C., et al., "Estimates of the Prevalence of Arthritis and Selected Musculoskeletal Disorders in the United States." *Arthritis and Rheumatism,* 41, 1998, pages 778–799.

14. Liang, M.H., and Fortin, R., "Management of Osteoarthritis of the Hip and Knee." *Journal of the American Medical Association,* 325 (2), 1991, pages 125–127.

15. Adams, M.E., "Cartilage Research and Treatment of Osteoarthritis." *Current Opinions in Rheumatology,* 4, 1992, pages 552–559.

Chapter 2: When Joints Go Bad

1. Buckwalter, J.A., et al., "Restoration of Injured or Degenerated Articular Cartilage." *Journal of the American Academy of Orthopaedic Surgeons,* 2(4), 1994, pages 192–201.

2. Caplan, A.I., "Cartilage." *Scientific American,* 251(l), October 1984, pages 84–97.

3. Buckwalter, J.A., et al., "Restoration of Injured or Degenerated Articular Cartilage." *Journal of the American Academy of Orthopaedic Surgeons,* 2(4), 1994, pages 192–201.

Chapter 3: New Hope for Beating Osteoarthritis

1. Mueller-Fassbender, H., Bach, G.L., Haase, W., et al., "Glucosamine Sulfate Compared to lbuprofen in Osteoarthritis of the Knee." *Osteoarthritis and Cartilage,* 2, 1994, pages 61–69.

2. Crolle, G., and D'Este, E., "Glucosamine Sulphate for the Management of Arthrosis: A Controlled Clinical Investigation." *Current Medical Research and Opinion,* 7(2), 1980, pages 104–109.

3. Manicourt, D.H., Poilvache, P., Nzeusseu, A., et al., "Serum Levels of Hyaluronan, Antigenic Keratan Sulfate, Matrix Metalloproteinase 3, and

Tissue Inhibitor of Metalloproteinases 1 Change Predictably in Rheumatoid Arthritis Patients Who Have Begun Activity after a Night of Bed Rest." *Arthritis and Rheumatism*, 42, 1999, pages 1861–1869.

4. Piperno, M., Reboul, P., Hellio le Graverand, M. P., et al., "Osteoarthritic Cartilage Fibrillation Is Associated with a Decrease in Chondrocyte Adhesion to Fibronectin." *Osteoarthritis and Cartilage*, 6, 1998, pages 393–399.

5. Meininger, M. A., Kelly, K. A., et al. "Glucosamine Inhibits Inducible Nitric Oxide Synthesis." *Biochemical and Biophysical Research Communications*, 279(1), 2000, pages 234–239.

6. Shikhman, A. R., Alaaeddine, A., and Lotz, M. K., "N-Acetylglucosamine Prevents IL-1-Mediated Activation of Chondrocytes." *Arthritis and Rheumatism*, 42(9 suppl.), 1999, page S381.

7. Dovanti, A., Bignamini, A. A., and Rovati, A. L., "Therapeutic Activity of Oral Glucosamine Sulphate in Osteoarthrosis: A Placebo-Controlled Double-Blind Investigation." *Clinical Therapeutics*, 3(4), 1980, pages 266–272.

8. Pujalte, J. M., Llavore, E. P., and Ylescupidez, E. R. "Double-Blind Clinical Evaluation of Oral Glucosamine Sulphate in the Basic Treatment of Osteoarthrosis." *Current Medical Research and Opinion*, 7(2), 1980, pages 110–114.

9. Cordoba, F., and Nimni, M. E., "Chondroitin Sulfate and Other Sulfates Containing Chondroprotective Agents May Exhibit Their Effects by Overcoming a Deficiency of Sulfur Amino Acids." *Osteoarthritis and Cartilage*, 11, 2003, pages 228–230.

10. Fenton, J. I., Chlebek-Brown, K. A., Peters, T. L., et al., "The Effects of Glucosamine Derivatives on Equine Articular Cartilage." *Osteoarthritis and Cartilage*, 8, 2000, pages 444–451; Karzel, K., Domenjoz, R., "Effect of Hexosamine Derivatives and Uronic Acid Derivatives on Glycosaminoglycan Metabolism of Fibroblast Cultures." *Pharmacology*, 5, 1971, pages 337–345.

11. Reginster, J. Y., Deroisy, R., Rovati, L. C., et al., "Long-Term Effects of Glucosamine Sulphate on Osteoarthritis Progression: A Randomised, Placebo-Controlled Clinical Trial." *Lancet*, 357, 2001, pages 247–248.

12. Pavelka, K., Gatterova, J., Olejarova, M., et al., "Glucosamine Sulfate Delays Progression of Knee Osteoarthritis: A 3-Year, Randomized, Placebo-Controlled, Double-Blind Study." *Archives of Internal Medicine,* 162, 2002, pages 2113–2123.

13. Dovanti, A., Bignamini, A. A., and Rovati, A. L., "Therapeutic Activity of Oral Glucosamine Sulphate in Osteoarthrosis: A Placebo-Controlled Double-Blind Investigation." *Clinical Therapeutics,* 3(4), 1980, pages 266–272.

14. Towheed, T., "Current Status of Glucosamine Therapy in Osteoarthritis." *Arthritis and Rheumatism,* 49(4), 2003, pages 601–604.

15. Tapadinhas, M. J., Rivera, I. C., and Bignamini, A. A., "Oral Glucosamine Sulphate in the Management of Arthrosis: Report on a Multicentre Open Investigation in Portugal." *Pharmatherapeutica,* 3(3), 1982, pages 157–168.

16. Fassbender, H. M., et al., "Glucosamine Sulfate Compared to Ibuprofen in Osteoarthritis of the Knee." *Osteoarthritis and Cartilage,* 2(1), 1994, pages 61–69.

17. Norman, M. R., "Evaluation of Glucosamine Sulfate Compared to Ibuprofen for the Treatment of Temporomandibular Joint Osteoarthritis: A Randomized Double Blind Controlled 3 Month Clinical Trial." *Journal of the American Medical Association,* 286(6), 2001, page 654.

18. Caplan, A. I., "Cartilage." *Scientific American,* October 1984, pages 84–97.

19. Conte, A., Volpi, N., Palmieri, L., et al., "Biochemical and Pharmacokinetic Aspects of Oral Treatment with Chondroitin Sulfate." *Arzneimittelforschung,* 45(8), 1995, pages 918–925.

20. Ronca, F., Palmieri, L., et al., "Anti-Inflammatory Activity of Chondroitin Sulfate." *Osteoarthritis and Cartilage,* 6(Suppl. A), 1998, pages 14–21.

21. Soldani, G., and Romagnoli, J., "Experimental and Clinical Pharmacology of Glycosaminoglycans (GAGs)." *Drugs in Experimental and Clinical Research,* 18(1), 1991, pages 81–85.

22. Conrozier, T., "Death of Articular Chondrocytes. Mechanisms and Protection" [French]. *Presse Medicin,* 27(36), 1998, pages 1859–1861.

23. Soldani, G., and Romagnoli, J., "Experimental and Clinical Pharmacology of Glycosaminoglycans (GAGs)," *Drugs in Experimental and Clinical Research,* 18(1), 1991, pages 81–85.

24. Nishikawa, H., Mori, I., and Umemoto, J., "Influences of Sulfated Glycosaminoglycans on Biosynthesis of Hyaluronic Acid in Rabbit Knee Synovial Membranes." *Archives of Biochemistry and Biophysics,* 240, 1985, pages 145–153; Videla Dorna, I., and Guerrero, R. C., "Effects of Oral and Intramuscular Use of Chondroitin Sulphate in Induced Equine Aseptic Arthritis." *Journal of Equine Veterinary Science,* 18, 1998, pages 548–550.

25. Hamon, V., "Effect of One Compound Structum® on Cytokines Secretion by Human Macrophages and PBMC." Pierre Fabre Laboratories—Internal Reports, 1997, pages 1–32.

26. Ronca, F., Palmieri, L., et al., "Anti-inflammatory Activity of Chondroitin Sulfate." *Osteoarthritis and Cartilage,* 6(Suppl. A), 1998, pages 14–21; Weyers, W., and Iseli, D., "Expériences pharmacologiques sur l'efficacité anti-philogistique de chondroitine sulfrique (Structum®)." *Therapie Woche Schweiz,* 3, 1987, pages 869–874.

27. Hardingham, T., "Chondroitin Sulphate and Joint Disease." *Osteoarthritis and Cartilage,* 6(Suppl. A), 1998, pages 3–5.

28. Lippiello, L., Woodward, J., Karpman, R., and Hammad, T. A., "In Vivo Chondroprotection and Metabolic Synergy of Glucosamine and Chondroitin Sulfate." *Clinical Orthopedics,* 381, 2000, pages 229–240.

29. McAlindon, T. E., LaValley, M. P., Gulin, J. P., and Felson, D. T., "Glucosamine and Chondroitin for Treatment of Osteoarthritis: A Systematic Quality Assessment and Meta-Analysis." *Journal of the American Medical Association,* 283(11), 2000, pages 1469–1475.

30. Michel, B., Vignon, E., et al., "Oral Chondroitin Sulphate in Knee OA Patients: Radiographic Outcomes of a 2-Year Prospective Study." *Osteoarthritis and Cartilage,* 9(suppl B), 2001, page S68.

31. Michel, B. A., Stucki, G., et al., "Retardation of Knee Joint Space Narrowing Through Chondroitin 4&6 Sulphate." *Arthritis and Rheumatism,* 48 (9 suppl), 2003, page S77.

32. Mazières, B., et al., "Le Chondroitin Sulfate dans le Traitement de la Gonarthrose et de la Coxarthrose." *Rev. Rheum. Mal Osteoartic,* 59(7–8), 1992, pages 466–472.

33. Conrozier, T., "Chondroitin Sulfates (CS 4&6): Practical Applications and Economic Impact" [French]. *Presse Medicin,* 27(36), 1998, pages 1866–1868.

34. Soroka, N. F., and Chyzh, K. A., "Clinical Efficiency and Pharmacoeco-
    nomical Evaluation of Treatment by Chondroitinsulphate (Structum®) in
    Patients with Primary Osteoarthritis (POA)." EULAR 2002 Annual
    Meeting, Stockholm, Sweden.

35. McAlindon, T. E., LaValley, M. P., Gulin, J. P., and Felson, D. T.,
    "Glucosamine and Chondroitin for Treatment of Osteoarthritis: A
    Systematic Quality Assessment and Meta-Analysis." *Journal of the
    American Medical Association*, 283(11), 2000, pages 1469–1475; Richy, F.,
    Bruyere, O., Ethgen, O., et al., "Structural and Symptomatic Efficacy of
    Glucosamine and Chondroitin in Knee Osteoarthritis: A Comprehensive
    Meta-Analysis." *Archives of Internal Medicine*, 163, 2003, pages 1514–1522.

36. Lippiello, L., Woodward, J., Karpman, R., and Hammad, T. A., "In Vivo
    Chondroprotection and Metabolic Synergy of Glucosamine and
    Chondroitin Sulfate." *Clinical Orthopedics*, 381, 2000, pages 229–240.

Chapter 4: ASU: Adding to the Arsenal

 1. S-Adenosyl-L-Methionine for Treatment of Depression, Osteoarthritis,
    and Liver Disease. Summary, Evidence Report/Technology Assessment:
    Number 64. AHRQ Publication No. 02-E033, August 2002. Agency for
    Healthcare Research and Quality, Rockville, MD. www.ahrq.gov/clinic/
    epcsums/samesum.htm.

 2. Lozano, Y. F., Mayer, C. D., et al, "Unsaponifiable Matter, Total Sterol and
    Tocopherol Contents of Avocado Oil Varieties." *Journal of the American Oil
    Chemists' Society*, 70(6), 1993, pages 561–565.

 3. Messina, M., and Barnes, S., "The Role of Soy Products in Reducing the
    Risk of Cancer." *Journal of the National Cancer Institute*, 83, 1991, pages
    541–546.

 4. Szczepanski, A., Dabrowska, H., and Moskalewska, K., "Piascledine in the
    Treatment of Scleroderma" [Polish]. *Przeglad Dermatologiczny*, 61(4), 1974,
    pages 525–527; Szczepanski, A., Dabrowska, H., and Moskalewska, K.,
    "Effect of Piascledine Treatment of Scleroderma" [Polish]. *Przeglad Derma-
    tologiczny*, 62(4), 1975, pages 555–558; Jarzab, G., "Piascledine in the Treat-
    ment of Parodontopathies" [Polish]. *Czasopismo Stomatologiczne*, 28(4),
    1975, pages 443–445.

 5. Nguyen, T. T., "The Cholesterol-Lowering Action of Plant Stanol Esters."
    Journal of Nutrition, 129, 1999, pages 2109–2112; Ling, W. H., and Jones,

P. J. H., "Dietary Phytosterols: A Review of Metabolism, Benefits and Side Effects." *Life Sciences,* 57, 1995, pages 195–206.

6. Kris-Etherton, P. M., Hecker, K. D., Bonanome, A., et al., "Bioactive Compounds in Foods: Their Role in the Prevention of Cardiovascular Disease and Cancer." *American Journal of Medicine,* 113(Suppl. 9B), 2002, pages 71S–88S.

7. Bouic, P. J., "Sterols and Sterolins: New Drugs for the Immune System?" *Drug Discovery Today,* 7(14), 2002, pages 775–778; Bouic, P. J., "The Role of Phytosterols and Phytosterolins in Immune Modulation: A Review of the Past 10 Years." *Current Opinion in Clinical Nutrition and Metabolic Care,* 4(6), 2001, pages 471–475.

8. Gerber, G. S., "Phytotherapy for Benign Prostatic Hyperplasia." *Current Urology Reports,* 3(4), 2001, pages 285–291.

9. Henrotin, Y. E., Labasse, A. H., Jaspar, J. M., et al., "Effects of Three Avocado/Soybean Unsaponifiable Mixtures on Metalloproteinases, Cytokines and Prostaglandin E2 Production by Human Articular Chondrocytes." *Clinical Rheumatology,* 17(1), 1998, pages 31–39.

10. Ibid.

11. Henrotin, Y. E., Sanchez, C., Deberg, M. A., et al., "Avocado/Soybean Unsaponifiables Increase Aggrecan Synthesis and Reduce Catabolic and Proinflammatory Mediator Production by Human Osteoarthritic Chondrocytes." *Journal of Rheumatology,* 30(8), 2003, pages 1825–1834.

12. Little, C. V., Parsons, T., and Logan, S., "Herbal Therapy for Treating Osteoarthritis (Cochrane Review)." In: *The Cochrane Library,* 2, 2001.

13. Lequesne, M., Maheu, E., Cadet, C., and Dreiser, R. L., "Structural Effect of Avocado/Soybean Unsaponifiables on Joint Space Loss in Osteoarthritis of the Hip." *Arthritis Care and Research,* 47(1) 2002, pages 50–58.

14. Appelboom, T., Schuermans, J., Verbruggen, G., Henrotin, Y., and Reginster, J. Y., "Symptoms Modifying Effect of Avocado/Soybean Unsaponifiables (ASU) in Knee Osteoarthritis: A Double Blind, Prospective, Placebo-Controlled Study." *Scandinavian Journal of Rheumatology,* 30(4), 2001, pages 242–247.

15. Maheu, E., Mazieres, B., Valat, J. P., et al., "Symptomatic Efficacy of Avocado/Soybean Unsaponifiables in the Treatment of Osteoarthritis of the

Knee and Hip: A Prospective, Randomized, Double-Blind, Placebo-Controlled, Multicenter Clinical Trial with a Six-Month Treatment Period and a Two-Month Followup Demonstrating a Persistent Effect." *Arthritis and Rheumatism,* 41(1), 1998, pages 81–91.

Chapter 5: The Arthritis Cure

1. Bolen, J., Helmick, C. G., Sacks, J. J., et al., "Adults Who Have Never Seen a Health-Care Provider for Chronic Joint Symptoms—United States, 2001." *Morbidity and Mortality Weekly Report,* 52(18), 2003, pages 416–419.

2. Fries, J. F., et al., "Running and the Development of Disability with Age." *Annals of Internal Medicine,* 121, 1994, pages 502–509.

3. Bunning, R. D., and Materson, R. S., "A Rational Program of Exercise for Patients with Osteoarthritis." *Seminars in Arthritis and Rheumatism,* 21(3), 1991, pages 33–43.

4. Felson, D. T., et al., "Weight Loss Reduces the Risk for Symptomatic Knee Osteoarthritis in Women: The Framingham Study." *Annals of Internal Medicine,* 116, 1992, pages 535–539.

5. Traut, E. F., and Thrift, C. B., "Obesity in Arthritis: Related Factors, Dietary Factors." *Journal of the American Geriatric Society,* 17, 1969, pages 710–717.

6. Moseley, J. B., O'Malley, K., Petersen, N. J., et al., "A Controlled Trial of Arthroscopic Surgery for Osteoarthritis of the Knee." *New England Journal of Medicine,* 347(2), 2002, pages 81–88.

7. Parsch, D., and Bru, T. H., "Replicative Aging of Human Articular Chondrocytes during Ex Vivo Expansion." *Arthritis and Rheumatism,* 46(11), 2002, pages 2911–2916.

8. Fox, S., and Fox, B. *Beyond Positive Thinking.* Carson, Calif.: Hay House, 1991, page 64.

Chapter 6: Choosing and Using Arthritis Supplements

1. Russell, A. S., Aghazadeh-Habashi, A., and Jamali, F., "Active Ingredient Consistency of Commercially Available Glucosamine Sulfate Products." *Journal of Rheumatology,* 29, 2002, pages 2407–2409.

2. Michel, B., Vignon, E., et al., "Oral Chondroitin Sulphate in Knee OA Patients: Radiographic Outcomes of a 2-Year Prospective Study." *Osteoarthritis and Cartilage,* 9(suppl. B), 2001, page S68.

3. Ibid.

4. Scroggie, D.A., Albright, A., and Harris, M.D., "The Effect of Glucosamine-Chondroitin Supplementation on Glycosylated Hemoglobin Levels in Patients with Type 2 Diabetes Mellitus: A Placebo-Controlled, Double-Blinded, Randomized Clinical Trial." *Archives of Internal Medicine,* 163(13), 2003, pages 1587–1590.

5. Reginster, J.Y., Deroisy, R., Rovati, L.C., et al., "Long-Term Effects of Glucosamine Sulphate on Osteoarthritis Progression: A Randomised, Placebo-Controlled Clinical Trial." *Lancet,* 357, 2001, pages 247–248. Lead author presentation postpublication.

6. Adebowale, A.O., Cox, D.S., Liang, Z., and Eddington, N.D., "Analysis of Glucosamine and Chondroitin Sulfate Content in Marketed Products and the Caco-2 Permeability of Chondroitin Sulfate Raw Materials." *Journal of the American Nutraceutical Association,* 3(1), 2000, pages 37–44.

7. *Consumer Reports,* January 2002.

8. Russell, A.S., Aghazadeh-Habashi, A., and Jamali, F., "Active Ingredient Consistency of Commercially Available Glucosamine Sulfate Products." *Journal of Rheumatology,* 29, 2002, pages 2407–2409.

Chapter 7: The Problem with Painkillers

1. Singh, G., "Recent Considerations in Nonsteroidal Anti-inflammatory Drug Gastropathy." *American Journal of Medicine,* 105(1B), 1998, pages 31S-38S; Wolfe, M., Lichtenstein, D., and Singh, G., "Gastrointestinal Toxicity of Nonsteroidal Anti-Inflammatory Drugs." *New England Journal of Medicine,* 340(24), 1999, pages 1888–1889.

2. Curhan, G.C., Willett, W.C., Rosner, B., and Stampfer, M.J., "Frequency of Analgesic Use and Risk of Hypertension in Younger Women." *Archives of Internal Medicine,* 162, 2002, pages 2204–2208.

3. Dedier, J., Stampfer, M.J., Hankinson, S.E., et al., "Nonnarcotic Analgesic Use and the Risk of Hypertension in U.S. Women." *Hypertension,* 40, 2002, pages 604–608.

4. Ruoff, G.E., "The Impact of Nonsteroidal Anti-Inflammatory Drugs on Hypertension: Alternative Analgesics for Patients at Risk." *Clinical Therapeutics,* 20, 1998, pages 376–387.

5. Bradley, J.D., et al., "Comparison of an Anti-Inflammatory Dose of Ibuprofen, an Analgesic Dose of Ibuprofen, and Acetaminophen in the Treatment of Patients with Osteoarthritis of the Knee." *New England Journal of Medicine,* 325, 1991, pages 87–91.

6. Sandler, D.P., Smith, J.C., Weinberg, C.R., et al., "Analgesic Use and Chronic Renal Disease." *New England Journal of Medicine,* 320, 1989, pages 1238–1243.

7. Garcia Rodriguez, L.A., and Hernandez-Diaz, S., "Relative Risk of Upper Gastrointestinal Complications among Users of Acetaminophen and Nonsteroidal Anti-Inflammatory Drugs." *Epidemiology,* 12, 2001, pages 570–576.

8. Kuffner, E.K., Dart, R.C., Bogdan, G.M., et al., "Effect of Maximal Daily Doses of Acetaminophen on the Liver of Alcoholic Patients: A Randomized, Double-Blind, Placebo-Controlled Trial." *Archives of Internal Medicine,* 161, 2001, pages 2247–2252.

9. Ostapowicz, G., Fontana, R.J., Schiodt, F.V., et al., "Results of a Prospective Study of Acute Liver Failure at 17 Tertiary Care Centers in the United States." *Annals of Internal Medicine,* 137, 2002, pages 947–954.

10. Bolesta, S., and Haber, S.L., "Hepatoxicity Associated with Chronic Acetaminophen Administration in Patients without Risk Factors." *Annals of Pharmacotherapy,* 36, 2002, pages 331–333.

11. Sandler, D.P., Smith, J.C., Weinberg, C.R., et al., "Analgesic Use and Chronic Renal Disease." *New England Journal of Medicine,* 320, 1989, pages 1238–1243.

12. Fored, C.M., Ejerblad, E., Lindblad, P., et al., "Acetaminophen, Aspirin, and Chronic Renal Failure." *New England Journal of Medicine,* 345, 2001, pages 1801–1808.

13. Williams, H.J., Ward, J.R., Egger, M.J., et al., "Comparison of Naproxen and Acetaminophen in a Two-Year Study of Treatment of Osteoarthritis of the Knee." *Arthritis and Rheumatism,* 36, 1993, pages 1196–1206.

14. Catella-Lawson, F., Reilly, M.P., Kapoor, S.C., et al., "Cyclooxygenase Inhibitors and the Antiplatelet Effects of Aspirin." *New England Journal of Medicine,* 345, 2001, pages 1809–1817.

15. Ding, C., "Do NSAIDs Affect the Progression of Arthritis?" *Inflammation*, 26, 2002, pages 139–142.

16. Rashad, S., Revell, P., Hemingway, A., et al., "Effect of Non-Steroidal Anti-Inflammatory Drugs on the Course of Osteoarthritis." *Lancet*, 2, 1989, pages 519–522.

17. Pelletier, J. P., "The Influence of Tissue Cross-Talking on OA Progression: Role of Nonsteroidal Antiinflammatory Drugs." *Osteoarthritis and Cartilage*, 7(4), 1999, pages 374–376; Dingle, J. T., "The Effects of NSAID on the Matrix of Human Articular Cartilages." *Zeitschrift für Rheumatologie*, 58(3), 1999, pages 125–129; Hugenberg, S. T., Brandt, K. D., and Cole, C. A., "Effect of Sodium Salicylate, Aspirin, and Ibuprofen on Enzymes Required by the Chondrocyte for Synthesis of Chondroitin Sulfate." *Journal of Rheumatology*, 20(12), 1993, pages 2128–2133; de Vries, B. J., van den Berg, W. B., and van de Putte, L. B., "Salicylate-Induced Depletion of Endogenous Inorganic Sulfate. Potential Role in the Suppression of Sulfated Glycosaminoglycan Synthesis in Murine Articular Cartilage." *Arthritis and Rheumatology*, 28(8), 1985, pages 922–929; Palmoski, M. J., and Brandt, K. D., "Effects of Some Nonsteroidal Antiinflammatory Drugs on Proteoglycan Metabolism and Organization in Canine Articular Cartilage." *Arthritis and Rheumatology*, 23(9), 1980, pages 1010–1020.

18. Stehlin, D., "How to Take Your Medicine—Nonsteroidal Antiinflammatory Drugs." *FDA Consumer*, June 1990, pages 33–34.

19. Silverstein, F. E., Faich, G., Goldstein, J. L., et al., "Gastrointestinal Toxicity with Celecoxib vs Nonsteroidal Anti-Inflammatory Drugs for Osteoarthritis and Rheumatoid Arthritis: The CLASS Study: A Randomized Controlled Trail. Celecoxib Long-Term Arthritis Safety Study." *Journal of the American Medical Association*, 284, 2000, pages 1247–1255.

20. Chan, F. K., Hung, L. C., Suen, B. Y., et al., "Celecoxib versus Diclofenac and Omeprazole in Reducing the Risk of Recurrent Ulcer Bleeding in Patients with Arthritis." *New England Journal of Medicine*, 347, 2002, pages 2104–2110.

21. Bombardier, C., Laine, L., Reicin, A., et al., "Comparison of Upper Gastrointestinal Toxicity of Rofecoxib and Naproxen in Patients with Rheumatoid Arthritis. VIGOR Study Group." *New England Journal of Medicine*, 343, 2000, pages 1520–1528.

22. Day, R., Morrison, B., Luza, A., et al., "A Randomized Trial of the Efficacy and Tolerability of the COX-2 Inhibitor Rofecoxib vs Ibuprofen in Patients with Osteoarthritis. Rofecoxib/Ibuprofen Comparator Study Group." *Archives of Internal Medicine,* 160, 2000, pages 1781–1787.

23. Geba, G. P., Weaver, A. L., Polis, A. B., et al., "Efficacy of Rofecoxib, Celecoxib, and Acetaminophen in Osteoarthritis of the Knee: A Randomized Trial." *Journal of the American Medical Association,* 287, 2002, pages 64–71.

24. Bombardier, C., Laine, L., Reicin, A., et al., "Comparison of Upper Gastrointestinal Toxicity of Rofecoxib and Naproxen in Patients with Rheumatoid Arthritis. VIGOR Study Group." *New England Journal of Medicine,* 343, 2000, pages 1520–1528.

25. Mukherjee, D., Nissen, S. E., and Topol, E. J., "Risk of Cardiovascular Events Associated with Selective COX-2 Inhibitors." *Journal of the American Medical Association,* 286, 2001, pages 954–959.

26. Ray, W. A., Stein, C. M., Daugherty, J. R., et al., "COX-2 Selective Non-Steroidal Anti-Inflammatory Drugs and Risk of Serious Coronary Heart Disease." *Lancet,* 360, 2002, pages 1071–1073.

Chapter 8: Exercise That *Helps*, Not Hurts

1. Gecht, M. R., et al., "A Survey of Exercise Beliefs and Exercise Habits Among People with Arthritis." *Arthritis Care and Research,* 9(2), 1996, pages 82–88.

2. Rock, M., "A Strong Case for Strength Training." *Arthritis Today,* 8(6), 1994, pages 45–50.

3. Miyaguchi, M., Kobayashi, A., et al., "Biochemical Change in Joint Fluid after Isometric Quadriceps Exercise for Patients with Osteoarthritis of the Knee." *Osteoarthritis and Cartilage,* 11, 2003, pages 252–259.

4. Bunning, R. D., and Materson, R. S., "A Rational Program of Exercise for Patients with Osteoarthritis." *Seminars in Arthritis and Rheumatism,* 21(3), 1991, pages 33–43.

5. Rock, M., "A Strong Case for Strength Training." *Arthritis Today,* 8(6), 1994, pages 45–50.

6. Morrow, S., "Take It in Stride: Walking Is Fun for Fall." *Arthritis Today,* 8(5), 1994, pages 59–61.

7. *Arthritis Information: Exercise and Your Arthritis.* Brochure No. 835-5455. Atlanta, Ga.: The Arthritis Foundation, January 1996.

8. McNeal, R. L., "Aquatic Therapy for Patients with Rheumatic Disease." *Rheumatic Disease Clinics of North America,* 16(4), 1990, pages 915–943.

9. "Stretching, the Truth," *UC Berkeley Wellness Letter,* November 1994, 11, pages 4–6.

Chapter 9: Healthy Eating Really Counts

1. Felson, D. T., Anderson J. J., Naimark A., et al., "Obesity and Knee Osteoarthritis. The Framingham Study." *Annals of Internal Medicine,* 109(1), 1988, pages 18–24.

2. Felson, D. T., Zhang, Y., Hannan, M. T., et al., "Risk Factors for Incident Radiographic Knee Osteoarthritis in the Elderly: The Framingham Study." *Arthritis and Rheumatism,* 40(4), 1997, pages 728–733.

3. Martin-Moreno, J. M., Willett, W. C., Gorgojo, L., et al., "Dietary fat, Olive Oil Intake and Breast Cancer Risk." *International Journal of Cancer,* 58, 1994, pages 774–780; Trichopoulou, A., Katsouyanni, K., Stuver, S., et al., "Consumption of Olive Oil and Specific Food Groups in Relation to Breast Cancer Risk in Greece." *Journal of the National Cancer Institute,* 87, 1995, pages 110–116.

4. De Lorgeril, M., Salen, P., et al., "Mediterranean Diet, Traditional Risk Factors, and the Rate of Cardiovascular Complications after Myocardial Infarction. Final Report of the Lyon Diet Heart Study." *Circulation,* 99, 1999, pages 779–785.

5. McAlindon, T. E., Jacques, P., Zhang, Y., et al., "Do Antioxidant Micronutrients Protect against the Development and Progression of Knee Osteoarthritis?" *Arthritis and Rheumatism,* 39, 1996, pages 648–656.

6. Travers, R. L., Rennie, G. C., Newnham, R. E., "Boron and Arthritis: The Results of a Double-Blind Pilot Study." *Journal of Nutritional Medicine,* 1, 1990, pages 127–132.

7. De Fabio, A., "Treatment and Prevention of Osteoarthritis." *Townsend Letter for Doctors,* February–March 1990, pages 143–148.

Chapter 10: Beating the Blues

1. O'Koon, M., "Out of the Dark." *Arthritis Today,* 9(1), January/February 1996, pages 34–40.

2. Ibid.

3. "Mental Disorders in America." NIH Publication No. 01-4584.

4. Keefe, F.J., Caldwell, D.S., Queen, K., et al., "Osteoarthritic Knee Pain: A Behavioral Analysis." *Pain,* 28, 1987, pages 309–321.

5. Murphy, H., Dickens, C., Creed, F., and Bernstein, R., "Depression, Illness Perception and Coping in Rheumatoid Arthritis." *Journal of Psychosomatic Research,* 46, 1999, pages 155–164.

6. S-Adenosyl-L-Methionine for Treatment of Depression, Osteoarthritis, and Liver Disease. Summary, Evidence Report/Technology Assessment: Number 64. AHRQ Publication No. 02-E033, August 2002. Agency for Healthcare Research and Quality, Rockville, MD. www.ahrq.gov/clinic/epcsums/samesum.htm.

7. McAlindon, T.E., Lavalley, M.P., and Felson, D.T., "Glucosamine and Chondroitin for Treatment of Osteoarthritis: A Systematic Quality Assessment and Meta-Analysis." *Journal of the American Medical Association,* 283, 2000, pages 1469–1475.

8. O'Koon, M., "Out of the Dark." *Arthritis Today,* 9(1), January/February 1996, pages 34–40.

9. Fries, J.F. *Arthritis: A Take Care of Yourself Health Guide.* Reading, Mass.: Addison Wesley, 1995, pages 238–239.

10. O'Koon, M., "Out of the Dark." *Arthritis Today,* 9(1), January/February 1996, pages 34–40.

11. Mondimore, E.M., *Depression: The Mood Disease.* Baltimore, Md.: The Johns Hopkins University Press, 1993.

12. Dexter, R., Brandt, K., "Distribution and Predictors of Depressive Symptoms of Osteoarthritis." *The Journal of Rheumatology,* 21(2), 1994, pages 279–286.

13. Creamer, P., Lethbridge-Cejku, M., and Hochberg, M.C., "Factors Associated with Functional Impairment in Symptomatic Knee Arthritis." *Rheumatology* 39, 2000, pages 490–496.

14. Creamer, P., Lethbridge-Cejku, M., and Hochberg, M.C., "Determinants of Pain Severity in Knee Osteoarthritis: Effect of Demographic and Psy-

chological Variables Using 3 Pain Measures." *Journal of Rheumatology*, 26, 1999, pages 1785–1792.

15. Orlock, C., "The Healing Power of Touch." *Arthritis Today* 8(6), November/December 1994, pages 34–37.

Chapter 11: You *Can* Prevent Osteoarthritis

1. Lavigne, P., Shi, Q., et al., "Modulation of IL-1β, IL-6, TNFα and PGE$_2$ by Pharmacological Agents in Explants of Membranes from Failed Total Hip Replacement." *Osteoarthritis and Cartilage*, 10(11), 2002, pages 898–904.

2. Felson, D. T., Anderson J. J., Naimark A., et al., "Obesity and Knee Osteoarthritis. The Framingham Study." *Annals of Internal Medicine*, 109(1), 1988, pages 18–24.

3. Felson, D. T., Zhang, Y., Hannan, M. T., et al., "Risk Factors for Incident Radiographic Knee Osteoarthritis in the Elderly: The Framingham Study." *Arthritis and Rheumatism*, 40(4), 1997, pages 728–733.

4. Sandmark H., Hogstedt, C., Lewold, S., and Vingard. E., "Osteoarthrosis of the Knee in Men and Women in Association with Overweight, Smoking, and Hormone Therapy." *Annals of the Rheumatic Diseases*, 58(3), 1999, pages 151–155.

5. Coggon, D., Reading, I., Croft, P., et al., "Knee Osteoarthritis and Obesity." *International Journal of Obesity and Related Metabolic Disorders*, 25(5), 2001, pages 622–627.

6. Flugsrud, G. B., Nordsletten, L., Espehaug, B., et al., "Risk Factors for Total Hip Replacement Due to Primary Osteoarthritis: A Cohort Study in 50,034 Persons." *Arthritis and Rheumatology*, 46(3), 2002, pages 675–682.

7. Felson, D. T., Zhang, Y., Anthony, M. J., et al., "Weight Loss Reduces the Risk for Symptomatic Knee Osteoarthritis in Women. The Framingham Study." *Annals of Internal Medicine*, 116(7), 1992, pages 535–539.

8. Selesnick, H., "Prevalence of Abnormal Findings on MRI in the Knees of Professional Basketball Players," Presentation at American Orthopedic Society for Sports Medicine, Sports Medicine and the NBA Conference, November 17, 2000, Miami Beach, Florida.

9. Jensen, M. C., Brant-Zawadzki, M. N., Obuchowski, N., et al., "Magnetic Resonance Imaging of the Lumbar Spine in People without Back Pain." *New England Journal of Medicine,* 331(2), 1994, pages 69–73.

10. Borenstein, D. G., O'Mara, J. W. Jr., Boden, S. D., et al., "The Value of Magnetic Resonance Imaging of the Lumbar Spine to Predict Low-Back Pain in Asymptomatic Subjects: A Seven-Year Follow-Up Study." *Journal of Bone and Joint Surgery,* 83 (A9), 2001, pages 1306–1311.

Index

About the Authors

Jason Theodosakis, M.D., M.S., M.P.H., F.A.C.P.M., also known as "Dr. Theo," is a practicing medical doctor. He is residency-trained, board-certified, and a Fellow in the specialty of preventive medicine. He is also fellowship-trained in Sports Medicine, a second specialty. His medical degree is from the University of Health Sciences/Chicago Medical School. He graduated summa cum laude with master's degrees in both Exercise and Sports Sciences and Public Health from the University of Arizona. His undergraduate education includes a double major (honors) in chemistry and biology from Florida International University.

Dr. Theodosakis divides his time between practicing clinical preventive medicine and sports medicine at the Canyon Ranch Medical Department, teaching, and volunteer activities. He is an assistant clinical professor at the University of Arizona College of Medicine and is the former director of the University's preventive medicine residency training program. He is on the oversight committee for the $16 million NIH trial on glucosamine and chondroitin and was named one of the world's 14 greatest doctors by Rodale Press.

The original edition of his treatment program, The Arthritis Cure, resulted in a major paradigm shift in the way arthritis is treated. The Arthritis Cure is estimated to save thousands of deaths per year by reducing the need for dangerous medicines and surgery. Now some 40 clinical trials support his theories and millions worldwide successfully follow his program. Dr. Theodosakis is committed to maintaining the integrity of the program's principles, including quality control and quality assurance in the dietary supplement industry.

Dr. Theo can be contacted through his Web site at www.drtheo.com.

Sheila Buff is the author or coauthor of many books on health and nutrition, including *The Good Fat, Bad Fat Counter, Dr. Atkins' Age-Defying Diet,* and *The Complete Idiot's Guide to Vitamins and Minerals.* She lives in New York's Hudson Valley.